I0407069

Nature's Painkillers:

A Guide to Natural Remedies from

U.K. Native Trees, Plants, and Fungi

Delyth Angharad Williams-Pryce

Disclaimer

This book intends to provide information about natural painkillers in the U.K.'s native trees, plants, and fungi. It is designed to help readers increase their understanding of the potential healing properties of the natural world around them. It is not a substitute for professional medical advice, diagnosis, or treatment.

Natural painkillers should always be under the guidance and supervision of a qualified healthcare provider. Readers need to consult their healthcare provider before beginning any new treatment to determine its appropriateness for their health needs. The author and publisher expressly disclaim responsibility for any adverse effects that may result from using or applying the information in this book.

Despite the author's efforts to provide accurate and up-to-date information, some of the material in this book may be subject to change based on further research or the evolution of medical knowledge. Therefore, readers are encouraged also to confirm the information with other sources.

Identifying and harvesting wild plants and fungi involve significant risks, including the risk of poisoning and death. The author and publisher are not responsible for any mishaps that may arise from using this guide. The reader is responsible for accurately identifying and safely using wild plants and fungi. By reading this book, you acknowledge and agree to use the information within at your own risk.

"Fungi are the grand recyclers of the planet and the vanguard species in habitat restoration." - Paul Stamets

Table of Contents

Introduction

$\mathbf{P}$ain is a common experience that affects many of us at some point. While over-the-counter and prescription medications are readily available, many people use natural remedies for pain relief.

We will discuss the benefits of using natural remedies for pain relief, including their potential to be effective and their low risk of side effects when used correctly. We will also provide an overview of the plants, trees, and fungi discussed in the following chapters.

Each plant, tree, or fungi will also include preparation, storage, and dosage information to ensure their safe use. Please note that while natural remedies can be effective for pain relief, they are not a substitute for medical advice. Therefore, it is essential to consult a healthcare professional before using any natural remedies.

Pain is an experience that can affect individuals to varying degrees, both physically and emotionally. Pain can occur in response to tissue damage, inflammation, or psychological factors and can be acute or chronic. While pharmacological interventions such as nonsteroidal anti-inflammatory drugs (NSAIDs) and opioids are commonly used for pain management, there is an increasing interest in using natural remedies for pain relief.

Natural remedies for pain relief have been used for centuries and continue to be used today by many individuals. These remedies include herbs, plants, trees, and fungi, which have been found to have analgesic and anti-inflammatory properties. Furthermore, natural remedies have fewer side effects than prescription medications, which is one of the reasons why individuals are seeking natural remedies for pain relief.

The use of natural remedies for pain relief has been recognised in many cultures, including traditional Chinese medicine, Ayurvedic medicine, and traditional European medicine. Many of the natural remedies in these cultures have been derived from plants, trees, and fungi native to the regions. In the U.K., there are several native plants, trees, and fungi that have been found to have potent analgesic properties.

This book will explore the natural painkillers in U.K. native trees, plants, and fungi. We will discuss their chemical constituents, mechanisms of action, and clinical applications. We will also provide an overview of the plants, trees, and fungi discussed in the following chapters.

The primary objective of this book is to provide readers with an understanding of natural painkillers and their potential applications for pain management. We will discuss the importance of preparation, storage, and dosage when using natural remedies to ensure their safe use.

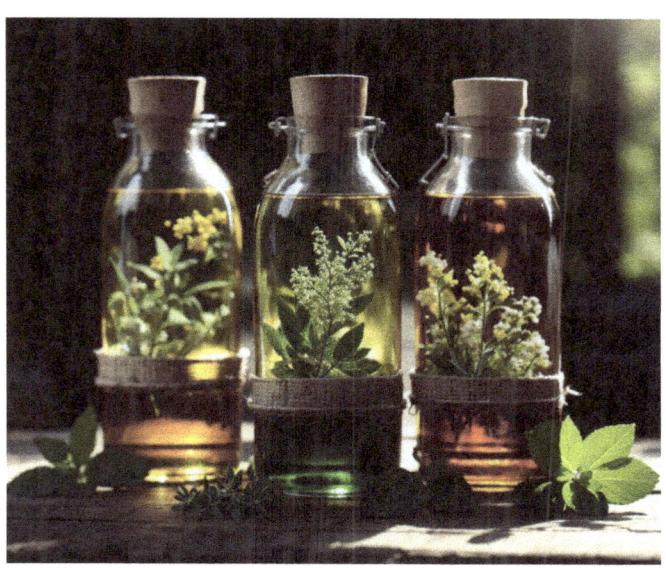

"The earth laughs in flowers." - Ralph Waldo Emerson

CHAPTER 1

Plants, Trees and Fungi - The Kingdom

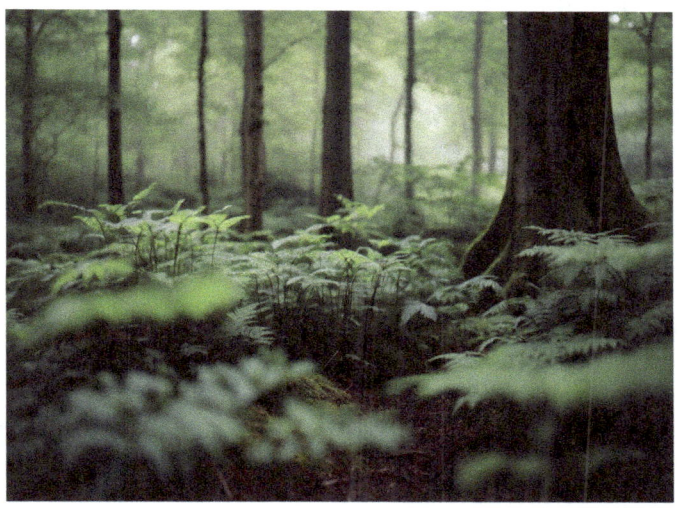

Deciphering the unique nuances among plants, trees, and fungi is like peeling the layers of an intriguing narrative, where each turn offers something fresh. Each layer, or in this case, each category, tells a unique story. Let's embark on this narrative.

The green expanse? The taxonomic and evolutionary context is akin to categorising characters in an epic tale. That's the kingdom Plantae, where mosses, ferns, and dashing flowers reside. Trees are the mighty protagonists, living amidst these other plants but standing tall and majestic. And fungi? They are the enigmatic entities, often misunderstood yet pivotal to the plot. Peek beneath the surface, and what do you find?

Cellular and physiological differences within the kingdom. Walls are not the kind you would lean on, but walls made of cellulose for plants and chitin for fungi. It's as if plants donned armour made of sunshine, water, and air while fungi weave their tapestry from the stories of other beings, decomposing, sharing, or sometimes parasitising.

Life's dance, the reproduction cycle, is a spectacle in itself. Reproductive variations and plants? They engage in intricate duets, sometimes alone, sometimes with partners, producing seeds that carry tales of pollen meeting ovules. Trees share these tales but have their twists - think of cones whispering secrets or seeds travelling with the wind.

Fungi, the versatile dancers, sometimes solo, sometimes with a partner, but always mesmerising, especially when they release spores, nature's confetti.

Life's not static, and it's an evolving saga. Plants and trees have aspirations; they aim for the skies, growing ceaselessly. Yet, fungi? They've mastered the art of 'enough', understanding when to expand and when to consolidate, with a strategy that's less about height and more about breadth.

In a Nutshell? One might think of them as characters in a grand play. Plants, including those stalwart trees and fungi, each have roles and tales that intertwine yet remain distinct. So next time you admire a tree, remember the saga it's a part of and the different narratives surrounding it.

"Plants give us oxygen for the lungs and for the soul." - Linda Solegato

CHAPTER 2

The Benefits of Natural Painkillers

The use of natural painkillers for pain management has several benefits. Firstly, natural remedies have fewer side effects than prescription medications. Natural painkillers are derived from plants, trees, and fungi and are usually less potent than synthetic drugs. Therefore, they are less likely to cause adverse effects, such as addiction, stomach ulcers, and liver damage associated with prescription painkillers.

Natural painkillers are often cheaper than prescription medications. While prescription medications can be expensive, natural remedies can be obtained relatively cheaply. This makes natural painkillers an attractive option for individuals who may not have access to or cannot afford prescription medications.

Natural remedies can be used with prescription medications to relieve pain. Many natural remedies have been found to enhance the effects of prescription medications and can be used to reduce the dosage required to manage pain. This can reduce the risk of side effects associated with prescription medications and improve overall pain management.

Natural painkillers have a long history of use in traditional medicine. Many of the natural remedies used in traditional medicine are effective in managing pain, and their safety has been established through centuries of use. This makes natural painkillers a reliable and trusted option for pain management.

Natural painkillers have a holistic approach to pain management. Natural remedies target the physical symptoms of pain and address the underlying causes of pain. This approach can help individuals relieve long-term pain by promoting overall health and well-being.

Overall, the benefits of natural painkillers make them a popular choice for individuals seeking alternative options for pain management. However, it is essential to note that natural remedies should not be used as a substitute for medical advice. Individuals should consult their healthcare provider before using any natural remedies.

Picking directly from Nature V's Health Shop, the Pros and Cons

Picking directly from nature, when done responsibly and knowledgeably, can offer various benefits compared to purchasing products from health shops.

Here's a breakdown

Freshness

Direct from Nature: Plants, herbs, and fungi picked fresh from their natural environment are often more vibrant and potent due to their freshness; this can translate into a higher nutritional and medicinal value.

Health Shop: Items in health shops, even if organic, might have been stored for extended periods, potentially decreasing their potency and freshness.

Cost

Direct from Nature: Foraging or picking your own can be cost-effective since you bypass the commercial chain of production, distribution, and retail.

Health Shop: Purchasing from a store involves costs related to production, transportation, storage, and retail markup.

Environmental Impact

Direct from Nature: Picking directly from nature can reduce the carbon footprint associated with transportation, packaging, and production.

Health Shop: Commercial production can have environmental consequences from farming practices, packaging, and long-distance transportation.

Connection to Nature

Direct from Nature: Engaging directly with the environment fosters a deeper connection to the land, enhancing mental well-being and grounding the individual.

Health Shop: Purchasing from a store can sometimes distance consumers from the source of their products, weakening the bond with nature.

Avoiding Additives and Preservatives

Direct from Nature: You get the product in its pure, unaltered state without added preservatives, fillers, or other chemicals.

Health Shop: Some commercial products might contain additives, preservatives, or other ingredients to extend shelf life or enhance appearance.

Knowledge and Skill Building

Direct from Nature: Foraging and picking your own requires knowledge about the local ecosystem, plant identification, and sustainable harvesting practices. This process can be educational and empowering.

Health Shop: Relying on store-bought products offers a different immersive learning experience.

Safety and Quality Control

Direct from Nature: There's a risk associated with picking your own, especially if you need to familiarise yourself with plant or fungi identification. Some plants and fungi have toxic look-alike.

Health Shop: Reputable health shops usually ensure their products meet specific safety and quality standards. There's less risk of misidentification or contamination. While picking directly from nature can offer numerous benefits like freshness, cost savings, and a deeper connection to the environment, it's essential to approach it responsibly. Knowledge about local ecosystems, proper identification skills, and sustainable harvesting practices are vital to ensure the safety and ecological integrity of the area. On the other hand, health shops provide convenience and a certain level of safety and standardisation but might need more freshness and potency of directly sourced items.

Natural Vs Synthetic Drugs

Natural painkillers offer several benefits compared to synthetic drugs. They are derived from plants, trees, and fungi that have pain-relieving properties and can be used to treat different types of pain, including chronic pain, acute pain, and neuropathic pain.

One of the most significant benefits of natural painkillers is that they are less likely to cause side effects than synthetic drugs. Synthetic drugs can have adverse effects on the liver, kidneys, and other organs and can be addictive. Natural painkillers are generally safer, as they are derived from natural sources and do not contain the same chemicals as synthetic drugs.

Natural painkillers are also often more affordable than synthetic drugs. Natural painkillers can be grown in gardens or harvested from the environment, making them easily accessible and inexpensive. This makes natural painkillers a practical option for those who cannot afford expensive synthetic drugs or cannot access them.

In addition to their pain-relieving properties, natural painkillers can also have additional therapeutic benefits, such as anti-inflammatory properties that can help alleviate pain caused by inflammation. In addition, natural painkillers, such as valerian root, can also have sedative effects that can help alleviate anxiety and promote relaxation.

Finally, natural painkillers are less likely to cause side effects, are often more affordable, and can have additional therapeutic properties. They can be sustainably harvested from the environment, making them more environmentally friendly than synthetic drugs. Synthetic drugs require large-scale manufacturing and production, which can have a significant environmental impact. On the other hand, natural painkillers can be harvested sustainably, preserving the environment and promoting biodiversity.

"The trees are our lungs, the rivers our circulation, the air our breath, and the earth our body." - Deepak Chopra

CHAPTER 3

Natural Painkillers from U.K. Native Trees, Plants, and Fungi

The U.K. is home to a wide range of native trees, plants, and fungi that have been found to have potent analgesic properties. These natural remedies have been used for centuries in traditional medicine and continue to be used today by individuals seeking natural pain relief. In this section, we will discuss some of the most common U.K. native trees, plants, and fungi that have analgesic properties.

Willow Bark (Salix spp): Willow bark has been used for centuries as a natural painkiller. The willow tree's bark contains salicin, a natural pain reliever and anti-inflammatory agent. Salicin is converted to salicylic acid in the body, an active ingredient in aspirin. Willow bark relieves pain associated with headaches, toothaches, and menstrual cramps.

Meadowsweet (Filipendula ulmaria):
Meadowsweet is a perennial herb used in traditional medicine as a natural pain reliever. The plant contains salicylic acid, a natural painkiller and anti-inflammatory agent. Meadowsweet effectively relieves pain associated with headaches, menstrual cramps, and joint pain.

St. John's Wort (Hypericum perforatum):
St. John's Wort is a herb used for centuries to treat various conditions, including pain. The herb contains hypericin and hyperforin, natural painkillers and anti-inflammatory agents. St. John's Wort effectively relieves pain associated with nerve damage, arthritis, and muscle pain.

Lavender Oil (topical) (Lavandula angustifolia):
Lavender oil is extracted from the flowers of the lavender plant. The oil is often used in aromatherapy to promote relaxation and improve sleep quality. It is also used as a natural remedy for headaches and other types of pain.

Wood Avens (Geum urbanum): Also known as herb Bennet, its root was traditionally used to treat various ailments, including toothaches. Wood Avens is a perennial herb commonly found in shaded woodlands, hedgerows, and gardens across the U.K. Sporting delicate yellow flowers and a distinctively clove-like scent, this herb has deep roots in natural medicine. Historically, it has been used as a remedy for digestive disorders fevers, and even as an antiseptic for wounds. The plant's reputed therapeutic benefits can be ascribed to its constellation of bioactive compounds, such as Eugenol, a compound found in cloves. It lends the plant its characteristic clove-like aroma. Eugenol possesses antiseptic, analgesic, and anti-inflammatory properties, making it valuable in addressing oral and digestive complaints.

Lesser Celandine (Ficaria verna): Traditionally, the plant was used to treat haemorrhoids, which is why it's sometimes called "pilewort." Lesser Celandine, often heralded as one of the first signs of spring, adorns the woodlands and damp meadows of the U.K. with its bright yellow, star-shaped flowers. This small perennial, a member of the buttercup family, has historically been used in herbal remedies to treat various ailments, notably haemorrhoids, for which it earned the nickname "pilewort." Its therapeutic properties can be attributed to a combination of bioactive compounds such as Protoanemonin and Ranunculin.

Mugwort (Artemisia vulgaris): Mugwort (Artemisia vulgaris), with its silvery-green leaves and tall, reddish-purple stems, is a perennial herb frequently found along roadsides, wastelands, and riverbanks throughout the U.K. Used to aid digestion, promote menstrual flow, and remedy parasitic worms, Mugwort is valued for its multifaceted applications and is utilised in natural medicine. The plant's diverse medicinal properties are due to its rich array of compounds, such as Thujone, Cineole, Camphor and Coumarins.

Ribwort Plantain (Plantago lanceolata): Native to the U.K. and common in meadows and lawns, ribwort plantain has been traditionally chewed or applied as a poultice to soothe toothaches and other pains. With its distinctive narrow, lance-shaped leaves and tall flower spikes, Ribwort Plantain is a common sight in meadows, pastures, and lawns across the U.K. This hardy perennial has been a staple in natural medicine, offering remedies for everything from respiratory complaints to skin ailments. Its efficacy as a medicinal plant is attributed to a wealth of bioactive compounds such as Mucilage and Iridoid Glycosides naturally present in the plant.

Couch Grass (Elymus repens): Traditionally used as a diuretic to treat urinary tract infections, its soothing properties might indirectly help with pain associated with such infections. Couch Grass, known as twitch grass or quackgrass, is a perennial grass species proliferating across fields, gardens, and open grounds in the U.K. While often branded as a weed by gardeners, its intricate underground rhizome system has been tapped into for its medicinal benefits for centuries. In natural medicine, couch grass rhizomes are prized for their diuretic properties, aiding in urinary tract health and relieving infections and inflammations of the urinary system. This beneficial effect is attributed to a rich blend of chemical compounds found in the plant, such as Mucilage and Agropyrene.

Cowslip (Primula veris): The flowers and roots of this plant were historically used to make sedative and pain-relieving concoctions. Cowslip graces the meadows and open woodlands of the U.K. with its cheerful clusters of yellow, bell-shaped flowers atop slender green stems. This charming perennial in traditional herbal medicine is known for its soothing and pain-relieving properties.

Glycosides, specifically primverin and primulaverin, have been identified in cowslip. While their exact roles in pain relief or inflammation are not well-defined, glycosides in other plants are known to have various medicinal properties. Its flowers and roots have been employed in concoctions to combat insomnia, headaches, and coughs.

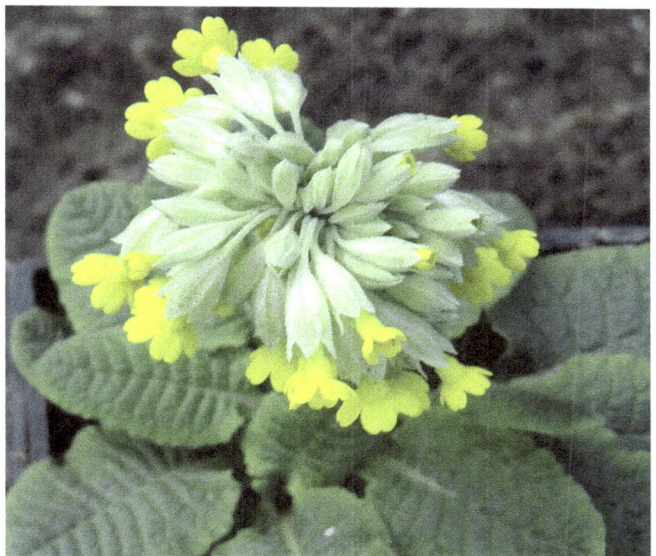

Cowslip

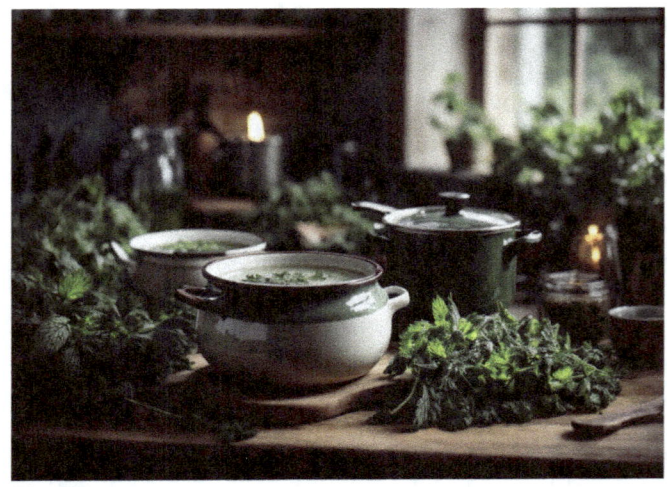

Nettle

Nettle (Urtica dioica): Nettle, often regarded with caution due to its stinging hairs, is a resilient herbaceous perennial native to the U.K. and many parts of the world. Its green, serrated leaves and tiny greenish-white flowers often grow abundantly in wild meadows and at the edge of woodlands. While an accidental brush against its leaves might result in a fleeting sting, nettle is rich in medicinal and nutritional virtues.

Historically, it has been harnessed to alleviate pain, especially in the context of arthritic conditions, thanks to its anti-inflammatory properties and, beyond pain relief, celebrated as a natural remedy for ailments ranging from allergies to anaemia. Rich in vitamins, minerals, and antioxidants, nettle leaves are often brewed into a nutritious tea or cooked similarly to spinach. Through its blend of health benefits and culinary applications, nettle defies its initial prickly reputation, emerging as a valuable asset in traditional medicine and the kitchen.

Hawthorn (Crataegus monogyna): Primarily known for its cardiovascular benefits, it has also been used to relieve pain. Hawthorn (Crataegus monogyna), a native tree to the U.K., is a sentinel of the countryside, easily recognisable by its dense thorny branches and clusters of delicate white or pink blossoms that herald the arrival of spring.

Beyond its beauty, hawthorn holds deep medicinal and cultural significance. Traditionally, various parts of the tree, especially its berries, leaves, and flowers, have been employed to address heart-related ailments. Rich in antioxidants and compounds such as Oligomeric Proanthocyanidins (OPCs) beneficial to cardiovascular health, hawthorn enhances blood circulation, regulates blood pressure, and supports overall heart function.

Bog Myrtle (Myrica gale): A deciduous shrub native to the wetlands and peat bogs of the U.K. and other parts of northern Europe, it is distinguished by its aromatic leaves and clusters of small yellow catkins. Various cultures cherish this plant for its multifaceted applications. Historically, Bog Myrtle was a crucial ingredient in brewing, imparting a unique flavour to beers before the widespread adoption of hops.

Beyond its culinary uses, it is esteemed for its medicinal properties, with traditional practitioners turning to it for pain relief and stomach ailments. Moreover, the fragrant leaves, when crushed, act as a natural deterrent to midges and other biting insects, making it a popular natural repellent. Bog Myrtle's enduring significance is a testament to nature's versatility, providing practical and therapeutic benefits.

Comfrey (Symphytum officinale): Traditionally used as a poultice for pain relief. Commonly referred to as "knitbone" or "bone-set," it is a perennial herb renowned for its deep purple, bell-shaped flowers and large, hairy leaves. Native to Europe, including the U.K., it has long held a revered spot in traditional herbal medicine. For generations, comfrey has been celebrated for its purported ability to accelerate the healing of bruises, sprains, and broken bones, a belief underscored by its folkloric names.

The plant's therapeutic properties are attributed to allantoin, which stimulates cell growth and repair. However, while its external applications are lauded, caution is advised regarding internal consumption due to certain alkaloids present in the plant that can be harmful if ingested in large amounts. As with many traditional remedies, comfrey's full spectrum of benefits and potential risks continues to be a subject of modern research and discussion.

Feverfew (Tanacetum parthenium): A perennial herb native to the U.K., is prominent in traditional herbal medicine. Historically prized for its distinctive lacy leaves and daisy-like flowers, its therapeutic significance primarily lies in its analgesic properties. Many have turned to feverfew over the centuries as a natural remedy for debilitating migraines and persistent headaches. This age-old reliance is rooted in the plant's ability to inhibit the release of serotonin and prostaglandins, which play roles in the onset of migraine episodes. While modern research continues to explore its benefits, feverfew remains a testament to nature's capacity to relieve some of the most common ailments.

Chanterelle Mushroom: Chanterelle mushrooms are a type of fungi that are found in the U.K. The mushrooms contain polysaccharides, which are natural anti-inflammatory agents. As a result, Chanterelle mushrooms are effective in relieving pain associated with arthritis and muscle pain.

These are just some of the many U.K. native trees, plants, and fungi with analgesic properties and in the following chapters, we will discuss these natural remedies in more detail, including their chemical constituents, mechanisms of action, clinical applications, and precautions to take when using them.

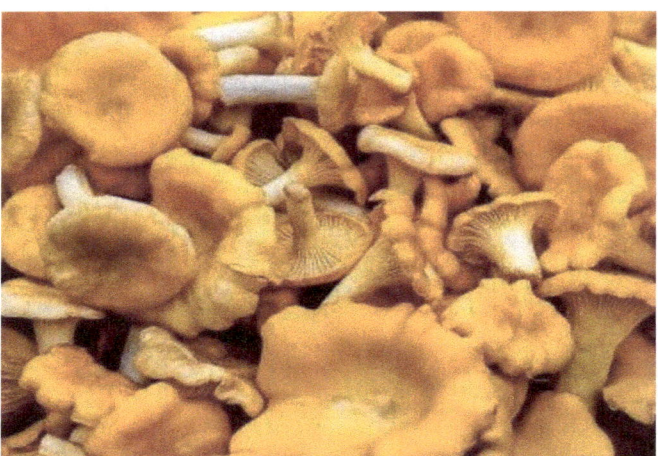

Chanterelle mushrooms

CHAPTER 4

Preparing and Storing Natural Painkillers

While natural painkillers can provide effective pain relief, knowing how to prepare and store them properly is vital to ensure their potency and safety. This chapter will discuss the best methods for organising and storing natural painkillers.

Preparation Methods: Several methods for preparing natural painkillers include making teas, tinctures, and poultices. The process depends on the type of natural painkillers used and the desired mode of administration.

Teas are a standard method of preparing natural painkillers. The plant material is steeped in hot water for several minutes to make tea. This method is often used for plants like meadowsweet and willow bark.

Tinctures are another popular method of preparing natural painkillers. Tinctures involve soaking the plant material in alcohol or vinegar to extract the active ingredients. This method is often used for herbs like St. John's Wort and Devil's Claw.

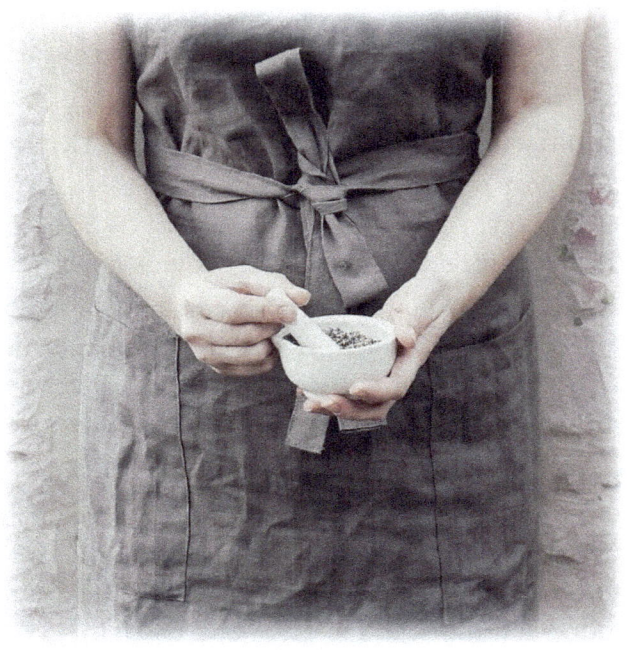

Poultices are used to apply natural painkillers directly to the affected area. The plant material is crushed and applied to the skin to make a poultice, often wrapped in a cloth or bandage. This method is often used for plants like comfrey and arnica.

Storage Methods: Proper storage of natural painkillers is essential for maintaining their potency and safety.

Here are some tips for storing natural painkillers:

- Store in a cool, dry place away from direct sunlight.

- Keep in airtight containers to prevent moisture and contamination.

- Label containers clearly with the plant's name, preparation method, and date of preparation.

- Keep out of reach of children and pets.

It is also important to note that natural painkillers can lose their potency over time. Therefore, it is recommended to use them within a few months of preparation and to discard any preparations that show signs of spoilage, such as mould or an unusual odour.

Dosage and Precautions: Following the recommended dosage and precautions are essential when using natural painkillers. Dosages can vary depending on the type of natural painkiller being used and the method of administration. It is necessary to consult with a healthcare professional before using natural painkillers, if you have any underlying medical conditions or are taking prescription medications. Some natural painkillers can have side effects and interact with other medications. For example, St. John's Wort can interact with certain antidepressants and birth control pills. Therefore, it is crucial to be aware of any potential interactions and to consult with a healthcare professional before using natural painkillers in combination with prescription medications.

In conclusion, proper preparation and storage of natural painkillers are essential for maintaining their potency and safety. Following the recommended dosage and precautions are necessary, and consult a healthcare professional before using natural painkillers.

"When we plant trees, we plant the seeds of peace and seeds of hope." - Wangari Maathai

A Simple Salve method, a simple step-by-step guide

Ingredients:

1 cup of oil (oil of your choice, such as sunflower oil or a combination of oils for differing properties)
1 ounce/29 grams of dried herbs or flowers
Cheesecloth or a fine-mesh strainer
A glass jar or container with a lid for storage.

Method:

- Start by decarboxylating your herbs. This process involves gently heating them to activate their beneficial compounds.

- Preheat your oven to 240°F (115°C).

- Spread the dried herbs evenly on a baking sheet lined with parchment paper and place them in the oven for 40-60 minutes or until they become slightly golden and fragrant.

- Once the herbs are decarboxylated, heat the oil in a double boiler over low heat. If you don't have a double boiler, you can create one by placing a heatproof bowl over a pot filled with a few inches of water. Ensure that the water doesn't touch the bottom of the bowl.

- Add the decarboxylated herbs to the oil and stir well to combine. Make sure all the herbs are fully immersed in the oil.

- Let the mixture simmer on low heat for at least 3 hours. This slow heating process allows the oil to fully infuse with the herbs, extracting their beneficial properties.

- After simmering, remove the mixture from heat and let it cool.

- Once the mixture has cooled down, strain it through a cheesecloth or fine-mesh strainer into a clean glass jar or container.

- Gently squeeze the herbs in the cheesecloth to extract as much oil as possible.

- Seal the jar tightly with a lid and store it in a cool, dark place for at least six months.

This extended period will allow the salve to mature and increase its potency fully.

After six months, strain the salve again to remove sediment or leftover herbs. Use a fresh cheesecloth or strainer for this step.

Your potent salve is now ready for use! Transfer it to smaller jars or tins for convenient application.

Remember, when using any home-made salve or herbal product, it's always a good idea to perform a patch test on a small area of your skin to check for any potential allergies or sensitivities.

To make the salve thicker for easier spreading, you can follow these additional steps:

- After straining the initial mixture of oil and herbs, return the infused oil to a clean double boiler or heatproof bowl.

- Heat the oil over low heat and add 1-2 tablespoons of beeswax pellets or grated beeswax per cup of infused oil. Beeswax acts as a natural thickening agent.

- Stir the mixture continuously until the beeswax has completely melted and combined with the oil.

- To test the consistency, you can take a small spoonful of the mixture and let it cool for a few minutes. If it's still too runny, add more beeswax in small increments until you achieve the desired thickness.

- Once satisfied with the consistency, remove the mixture from heat and let it cool slightly.

- Pour the salve into clean, sterilised jars or tins and allow it to cool completely. As it cools, it will solidify and thicken further.

- Once cooled, seal the containers with lids and store them in a cool, dark place for future use. By adding beeswax, you can customise the thickness of your salve according to your preferences. Just remember to gradually add the beeswax, as a little goes a long way, and you can constantly adjust it if needed.

Ingredients native to the U.K. and widely used in the past include:

Beeswax is a natural wax produced by bees and is commonly used in skincare products as a thickening agent and emollient. It adds a protective barrier to the skin and helps retain moisture.

Calendula, also known as marigold, is a flowering plant native to Europe. It is often used in skincare products due to its soothing and healing properties. Calendula extract or infused oil can be added to your salve mixture for its skin-calming benefits.

Rosehips are the fruit of wild rose plants and can be found in the U.K. Rosehip oil is rich in antioxidants and essential fatty acids, making it beneficial for moisturising, rejuvenating, and improving the appearance of scars and wrinkles.

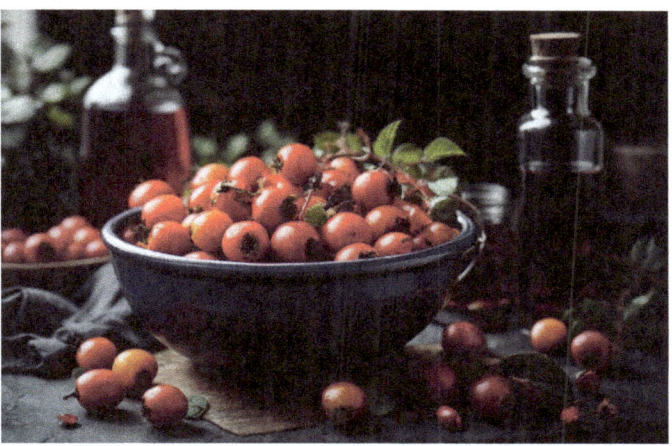

Rosehip

These native or locally available ingredients can provide similar properties and benefits to cocoa butter, allowing you to create a nourishing salve using local resources. Rosehip seed oil is extracted from the seeds of wild rose bushes. It is high in vitamins, antioxidants, and essential fatty acids, making it beneficial for skin rejuvenation and hydration. These oils can usually be found in health food stores, online retailers, or speciality cosmetic ingredient suppliers in the U.K.

Raspberry seed oil is rich in antioxidants and essential fatty acids. It is known for its hydrating and firming effects on the skin.

Animal fats can also be used for skin care and would have been the primary fats (oils) used in the past. However, it's important to note that animal fats are not typically sold as stand-alone oils for cosmetic use.

Some common animal fats include Tallow, which is rendered beef or mutton fat. It has historically been used in soap-making and skincare products due to its moisturising properties. Lard is rendered pork fat, commonly used in cooking and baking. It can also be used for skincare, as it is a rich source of moisturising fatty acids.

Rapeseed oil and Sunflower oil are commonly used in cooking and skincare. Rapeseed oil, also known as canola oil, is derived from the seeds of the rapeseed plant. It is a versatile oil with a mild flavour that can be used for frying, baking, and salad dressings. Rapeseed oil is also used in skin care products due to its moisturising and nourishing properties.

Sunflower oil is extracted from the seeds of the sunflower plant. Sunflower oil is also used in skin care products due to its light texture and moisturising benefits.

Rapeseed and sunflower oils are considered healthy cooking oils as they are low in saturated fats and monounsaturated and polyunsaturated fats. They are also a good source of vitamin E, an antioxidant that helps protect the body's cells from damage. When using these oils for skincare, choosing cold-pressed or organic options is essential to ensure the highest quality and purity.

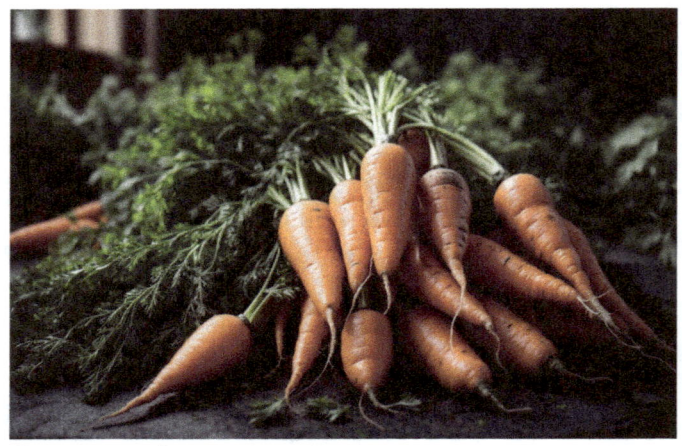

Carrot

Carrot oil can also be used in various applications. Carrot oil is derived from the seeds or roots of carrots and is known for its nourishing and rejuvenating properties. It is rich in vitamins A, E, and beta-carotene, which benefit the skin and hair.

Carrot oil is often used in skincare products due to its moisturising and anti-ageing effects. It can help improve skin tone, reduce the appearance of scars and wrinkles, and promote a healthy complexion.

Carrot oil is also believed to have antioxidant properties, helping to protect the skin from free radicals and environmental damage.

Some people also use carrot oil as a natural sunscreen due to its high beta-carotene content, although it should differ from traditional sun protection methods.

It's important to note that carrot oil is typically used as a carrier and is often diluted with other oils or ingredients before use. Undiluted carrot oil may be too potent and cause skin irritation in some individuals. As with any new skincare or haircare product, it's always recommended to do a patch test before applying it to a larger area.

The double heat method, also known as the double boiler method, is commonly used when making home-made infused oils. However, the specific method used to make carrot oil can vary.

- To make carrot oil using the double heat method, you typically start by finely grating or chopping fresh carrots. Then, place the grated or chopped carrots in a heat-resistant container, such as a glass jar or a stainless steel pot.

- Next, you would add a carrier oil of your choice or another vegetable oil to cover the carrots completely.

- The container with the carrots and oil is then placed in a larger pot filled with water. Heat is applied to the larger pot, creating a gentle and indirect heat source for the container with the carrots and oil.

- The water in the larger pot should be brought to a simmer, and the carrot and oil mixture should be heated for several hours, allowing the beneficial properties of the carrots to infuse into the oil.

It's essential to monitor the water level in the larger pot and ensure it doesn't completely evaporate, as this can cause the container with the carrot and oil mixture to overheat or even catch fire. It is recommended to use a heat-resistant container and to keep a close eye on the process throughout.

After the desired amount of time, the infused oil can be strained to remove the carrot solids, leaving behind the carrot oil. The strained carrot oil can then be stored in a clean, airtight container for later use. It's worth noting that there are other methods to make carrot oil, such as using a slow cooker or a hot infusion method. The choice of technique may depend on personal preference and equipment.

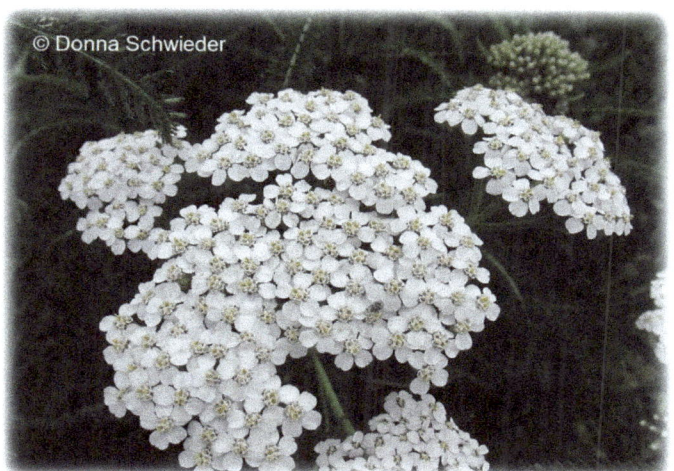

Yarrow

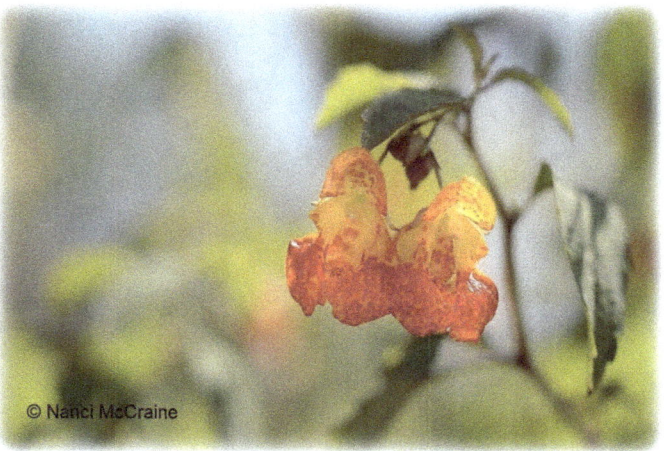

Jewelweed

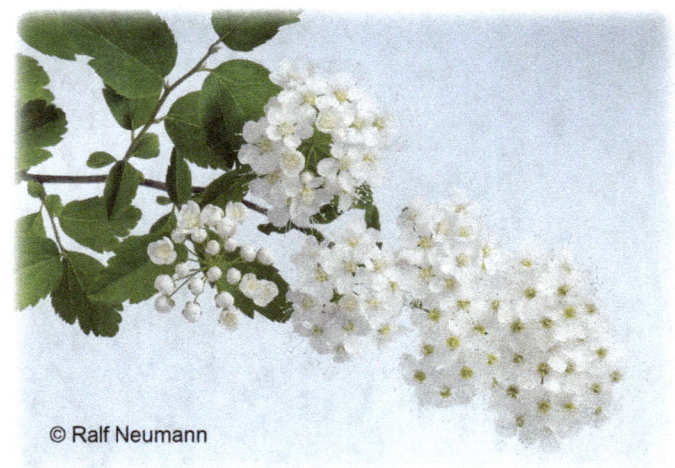

© Ralf Neumann

Meadowsweet

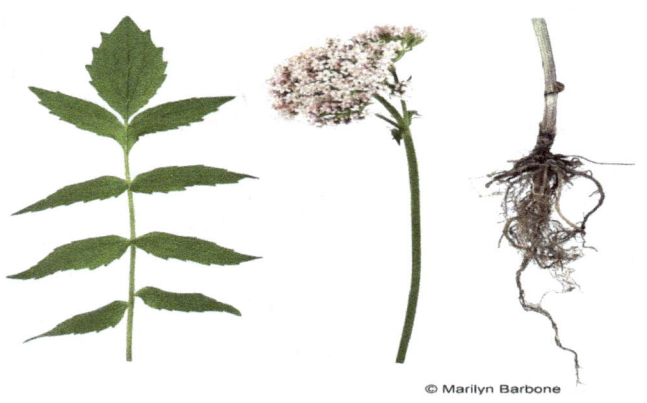

© Marilyn Barbone

Valerian Root

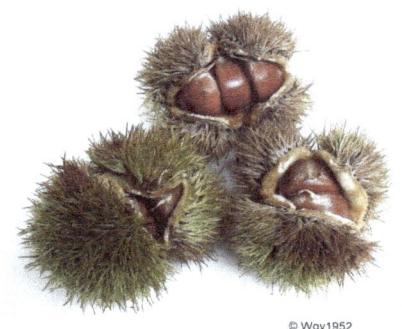

© Wgy1952

*Sweet Chestnut (edible) with less amount of Aescin. Horse Chestnut is often mistaken for Sweet Chestnut and has larger amounts of Aescin and is considered toxic.

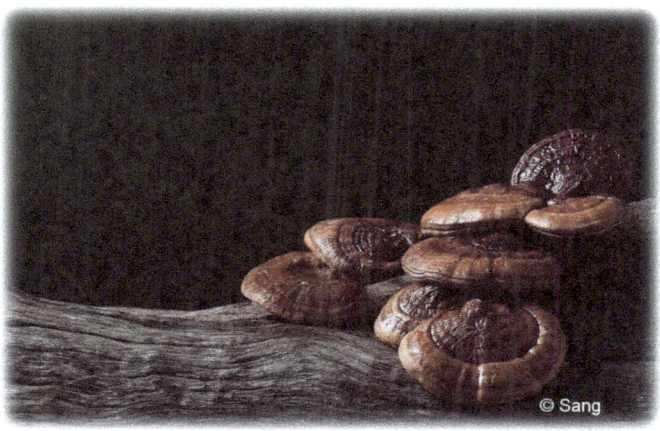

© Sang

Reishi mushrooms

CHAPTER 5

Chemical Constituents of Natural

Painkillers

Natural painkillers contain a variety of chemical constituents that are responsible for their pain-relieving properties. Understanding the chemical components of natural painkillers can help us understand how they work and how they can be used to treat different types of pain.

One group of chemical constituents found in many natural painkillers is called alkaloids. Alkaloids are nitrogen-containing compounds that are often bitter-tasting and have potent physiological effects. In addition, many alkaloids found in natural painkillers have analgesic properties and can be used to relieve pain. For example, opium poppy (Papaver somniferum) contains several alkaloids, including morphine and codeine, which are potent pain relievers.

Another group of chemical constituents found in natural painkillers are terpenes. Terpenes are volatile organic compounds responsible for many plants' distinctive smells and flavours. Many terpenes have pain-relieving properties and can be used to treat different types of pain. For example, the terpene beta-caryophyllene, found in black pepper and several other plants, has been shown to have analgesic effects.

Flavonoids are another group of chemical constituents found in many natural painkillers. Flavonoids are pigments that give many plants their bright colours and have various physiological effects. Some flavonoids have anti-inflammatory and analgesic properties and can be used to treat pain. For example, the flavonoid quercetin, found in many fruits and vegetables, has been shown to have analgesic and anti-inflammatory effects.

Essential oils are another group of chemical constituents found in many natural painkillers. Essential oils are volatile compounds responsible for many plants' characteristic smells. Many essential oils have pain-relieving properties and can be used to treat different types of pain. For example, the lavender essential oil has been shown to have analgesic effects and can be used to treat pain caused by headaches and muscle tension.

Phenolic compounds play a substantial role in various natural pain relievers. Its presence in essential oils from plants like clove, cinnamon, basil, and bay leaf underscores its widespread utility in analgesic formulations. The phenolic structure of Eugenol is pivotal for its anti-inflammatory and analgesic properties. It works by obstructing specific enzymes that contribute to inflammation and pain perception within the body.

Eugenol is commonly employed in dental settings as a topical analgesic, relieving toothaches and gum pain and efficiently numbs soft tissues. Phenol enables its therapeutic benefits, including anti-inflammatory and antibacterial actions.

Despite its various uses, the administration of Eugenol requires cautious attention to dosage and application to prevent potential irritation and other adverse reactions. The exploration of Eugenol's capacity to alleviate other pain and inflammatory conditions continues, highlighting the importance of its phenolic characteristics in pain management.

The glucoside compound Ranunculin is a precursor to protoanemonin in plants, particularly in the Ranunculaceae (buttercup) family. It is a non-toxic compound, but when the plant is damaged, ranunculin is hydrolysed enzymatically to produce the toxic compound protoanemonin. The chemical conversion involves breaking a glycosidic bond and a rearrangement that leads to the lactone structure of protoanemonin.

The specific chemical structure of ranunculin involves a glucose moiety bound to a compound that forms protoanemonin upon hydrolysis and rearrangement. Understanding the chemical pathway from ranunculin to protoanemonin is essential as it elucidates the toxicity mechanism in the Ranunculaceae family plants, highlighting the transformation from a non-toxic to a toxic compound upon plant damage. This knowledge is crucial for safely handling and using these plants, whether in horticulture, herbal medicine, or other applications.

To plants with analgesic properties, ketones, including specific types such as ketone esters, play a substantial role in contributing to the medicinal properties of various botanical species. Some plants produce ketone-containing compounds that have been explored for their potential analgesic (pain-relieving) and anti-inflammatory effects.

Particular ketones can interact with biological pathways in the human body to mitigate pain and inflammation, offering a natural avenue for pain management. For instance, some essential oils rich in ketones have been used in traditional medicine practices to alleviate pain and inflammation. The ketone functional group within these compounds may modulate various biochemical pathways, such as inhibiting the synthesis of inflammatory molecules or interacting with receptors involved in pain perception. However, it is crucial to approach plant-derived ketone compounds cautiously, ensuring proper dosage and consideration of potential side effects. Not all ketones are benign, and their results vary widely depending on their specific chemical structures and biological contexts.

In conclusion, natural painkillers contain a variety of chemical constituents that are responsible for their pain-relieving properties. Alkaloids, terpenes, flavonoids, and essential oils are just a few examples of the chemical components found in natural painkillers. Understanding the chemical constituents of natural painkillers can help us understand how they work and how they can be used to treat different types of pain.

CHAPTER 6

The Classification and differentiation of plants, trees, and fungi

The Classification and differentiation of plants, trees, and fungi are expounded from a morphological, physiological, reproductive, and evolutionary standpoint. This analysis will delineate the primary distinctions between these three categories.

Taxonomic and Evolutionary Context

Plants: All plants belong to the kingdom Plantae. They are multicellular eukaryotes that, for the most part, produce their food through the process of photosynthesis. This kingdom encompasses many organisms, including mosses, ferns, conifers, and flowering plants.

Trees: Trees are not a separate taxonomic group; instead, they are a subset of plants. Trees are typically defined as woody perennial plants, often with a single main stem or trunk, supporting branches and leaves. They can be found within several plant groups, including conifers (like pine trees) and angiosperms (like oak trees).

Fungi: Fungi belong to the kingdom Fungi and are distinct from plants. They are also multicellular eukaryotes but differ in cellular and metabolic aspects. Historically, fungi are classified under the Plant Kingdom due to some superficial similarities. Still, molecular studies have placed them in their own kingdom, more closely related to animals than plants.

Cellular and Physiological Differences

Cell Wall Composition: Plants primarily have cell walls made of cellulose, whereas fungi have chitin, a polymer also found in the exoskeletons of insects and other arthropods.

Nutritional Mode

Plants are autotrophs, synthesising their food via photosynthesis using sunlight, carbon dioxide, and water. Fungi, on the other hand, are heterotrophs. They decompose and absorb organic matter, making them either saprophytic, parasitic, or mutualistic.

Reproductive Variations

Plants: Plant reproduction can be both sexual (involving the formation and fusion of gametes) and asexual (like budding, fragmentation, or vegetative reproduction). Higher plants reproduce sexually by producing flowers which house the reproductive organs. Pollination and fertilisation then lead to seed formation.

Trees: A subset of plants, trees possess a similar reproductive strategy. However, trees' size, longevity, and woody nature have led to some unique adaptations in their reproductive methods, such as producing hard seeds, cones, or specialised dispersal mechanisms.

Fungi: Fungal reproduction is complex, involving both sexual and asexual methods. They reproduce asexually through spores, budding, or fragmentation. Sexual reproduction typically consists of the fusion of specialised sexual structures, leading to the production of spores.

Growth and Development

Plants and Trees: Both display indeterminate growth, meaning they can continue growing as long as they live, conditions permitting. Their growth is primarily through the activity of meristematic tissue in regions like the root and shoot tips.

Fungi: Fungi exhibit determinate growth, where the hyphal tips grow and extend into the substrate. Once a particular mycelium has colonised a substrate, its growth usually stops. Unlike plants, fungi do not have differentiated tissues or vascular systems.

While there are superficial similarities between plants (including trees) and fungi, such as their stationary nature and growth forms, these groups fundamentally differ in taxonomy, cellular structure, physiology, and reproductive strategies. Trees, being a category within the plant kingdom, share the overarching characteristics of plants but have specific adaptations suited to their more significant, perennial, and woody nature.

Neural Network of Earth

Mycelium as Earth's Neural Network

Mycelium, the vegetative part of fungi, forms vast underground networks that connect plants and trees. Paul Stamets, a renowned mycologist, often likens this to Earth's "neural network." Recent research suggests that trees and plants can communicate and exchange nutrients via these mycorrhizal networks, emphasising the interconnectedness of life.

Humans and the Earthly Network

From a holistic perspective, humans are also connected to this network. We can tap into this vast communication and energy system by respecting, preserving, and engaging with nature. The act of walking barefoot on the Earth, for instance, is seen by some as a way to "ground" one's energy and connect with the Earth's frequencies.

While modern science provides insight into the chemical and physiological interactions between humans and the natural world, traditional and holistic perspectives offer a more profound, energetic understanding. The idea is that by aligning with the energies and frequencies of native plants, trees, and fungi, humans can achieve greater harmony, health, and well-being.

Mycorrhizal Network

An Overview: A mycorrhizal network, often referred to as the **"Wood Wide Web"**, is a symbiotic association between the mycelium of fungi and the roots of plants. The term "mycorrhiza" itself is derived from the Greek words "mykes", meaning fungus and "rhiza" meaning root.

The mycorrhizal network is intricate and plays a vital role in forest ecosystems, as it facilitates the exchange of nutrients and signalling compounds between plants and fungi.

Here are the primary components and functions

Nutrient Exchange: Fungi, in general, are decomposers, breaking down organic matter in the soil into simpler substances. The fungus provides essential nutrients like phosphorus and nitrogen to the plant through the mycorrhizal relationship. In return, the plant provides the fungus with carbohydrates (sugars) that it produces via photosynthesis.

Signal Transmission: Beyond mere nutrient exchange, there's evidence suggesting that mycorrhizal networks allow plants to communicate with each other. This communication can involve alerting neighbouring plants of pest attacks, transferring carbon to neighbouring plants, or even influencing the growth rates of neighbouring plants.

Types of Mycorrhizae

There are several types of mycorrhizal associations, with the two most common being:

Ectomycorrhizae: The fungal mycelium envelops the root but doesn't penetrate individual root cells.

Endomycorrhizae (or arbuscular mycorrhizae): The fungal mycelium penetrates the root cells.

Ecological Importance: Mycorrhizal networks enhance plant survival by increasing their access to water and nutrients, especially in nutrient-poor soils. They also play a role in soil structure stabilisation and carbon storage.

Interplant Communication: Research, as previously mentioned, suggests that mycorrhizal networks enable plants to share resources, stabilising the plant community and offering mutual aid during stress.

In summary, the mycorrhizal network is a crucial ecological component that facilitates nutrient exchange between plants and fungi and plays an unexpected role in interplant communication and cooperation.

A foundational figure in this study area is Dr. Suzanne Simard, a University of British Columbia professor. Dr. Simard and her colleagues have published numerous articles on this topic.

For instance, Simard, S. W., Perry, D. A., Jones, M. D., Myrold, D. D., Durall, D. M., & Molina, R. (1997). Net transfer of carbon between ectomycorrhizal tree species in the field. Nature, 388(6642), 579-582.

Simard and her team demonstrated the net carbon transfer between plant species connected by a shared mycorrhizal network in this study.

"He that plants trees loves others besides himself." - Thomas Fuller

CHAPTER 7

Natural Analgesics: Mechanisms, Endocannabinoid Interactions, and Therapeutic Implications

Mechanisms of Action of Natural Painkillers

Natural painkillers work in a variety of ways to relieve pain. Understanding the mechanisms of action of natural painkillers can help us understand how they work and how they can be used to treat different types of pain.

One of the main mechanisms of action of natural painkillers is through their interactions with opioid receptors in the brain and spinal cord. Opioid receptors are proteins found in the nervous system and are responsible for mediating the effects of opioid drugs.

In addition, many natural painkillers contain alkaloids, such as morphine and codeine, which are agonists at opioid receptors and can produce potent pain relief.

Another mechanism of action of natural painkillers is through their interactions with the Endocannabinoid system. The Endocannabinoid system is a complex system of neurotransmitters and receptors regulating pain, mood, and other physiological processes. For example, many natural painkillers contain terpenes and other compounds that are agonists at cannabinoid receptors and can produce pain relief.

Natural painkillers can also work by inhibiting the production of inflammatory mediators such as prostaglandins and cytokines. Inflammation is a normal response to injury or infection, but chronic inflammation can contribute to pain and other pathological conditions. Many natural painkillers contain flavonoids and other compounds that have anti-inflammatory properties and can reduce pain by inhibiting the production of inflammatory mediators.

Natural painkillers can work by affecting the transmission of pain signals in the nervous system. Many natural painkillers contain essential oils and other compounds that can modulate the activity of neurotransmitters and channels involved in pain signalling. For example, the lavender essential oil has been shown to inhibit the release of the neurotransmitter glutamate, which is involved in pain signalling.

In conclusion, natural painkillers work in various ways to relieve pain. Opioid receptor activation, cannabinoid receptor activation, inhibition of inflammatory mediators, and modulation of pain signalling are just a few of the mechanisms of action of natural painkillers. Understanding these mechanisms of action can help us understand how natural painkillers work and how they can be used to treat different types of pain.

The Endocannabinoid system (ECS)

The Endocannabinoid system (ECS) is a complex biological system that regulates various physiological processes, including pain, appetite, mood, and immune function. It is named after the plant cannabis, which has been used for thousands of years for its medicinal and psychoactive properties. However, the ECS was discovered relatively recently in the 1990s, and its importance in human health is still being explored.

The ECS comprises three main components:

Endocannabinoids, receptors, and enzymes.

Endocannabinoids are naturally occurring compounds similar in structure to the cannabinoids found in cannabis. The primary Endocannabinoids are anandamide and 2-arachidonoylglycerol (2-AG), produced on demand in response to various stimuli.

The receptors of the ECS are found throughout the body, including in the brain, nervous system, immune system, and other organs. The two primary receptors are the CB1 receptor, primarily found in the brain and nervous system, and the CB2 receptor, primarily in the immune system and other peripheral tissues. Endocannabinoids bind to these receptors, producing a range of physiological effects.

The enzymes of the ECS are responsible for breaking down Endocannabinoids after they have fulfilled their role.

There are two main enzymes: fatty acid amide hydrolase (FAAH), which breaks down anandamide, and monoacylglycerol lipase (MAGL), which breaks down 2-AG.

The ECS plays a crucial role in maintaining homeostasis, or balance, in the body. It is involved in regulating pain, inflammation, appetite, and metabolism, as well as mood and stress responses. In addition, the ECS has been implicated in controlling various diseases, including epilepsy, multiple sclerosis, and chronic pain.

One of the most well-known effects of the ECS is its role in the psychoactive effects of cannabis. THC, the primary psychoactive compound in cannabis, binds to CB1 receptors in the brain, producing a range of influences, including euphoria, relaxation, and altered perception. However, the ECS is involved in many other processes beyond the psychoactive effects of cannabis.

There is ongoing research into the potential therapeutic applications of targeting the ECS. For example, drugs targeting the ECS may help treat chronic pain, inflammation, and anxiety disorders. However, potential risks are also associated with targeting the ECS, particularly with long-term use of THC or other cannabinoids.

The Endocannabinoid system is a complex and vital biological system that regulates various physiological processes. While much is still unknown about the ECS, ongoing research is likely to uncover new insights into its role in human health and disease.

Clinical Applications of Natural Painkillers

Natural painkillers have been used for centuries to treat pain and other ailments. While modern medicine has provided us with a wide range of pain-relieving drugs, natural painkillers are still widely used and are gaining more attention for their potential clinical applications.

One of the main clinical applications of natural painkillers is treating chronic pain. Chronic pain is a complex and often difficult-to-treat condition that can significantly impact a person's quality of life. Many natural analgesics, such as willow bark and devil's claw, in clinical trials effectively reduce chronic pain. As a result, they have often been considered a safer alternative to prescription opioids, which can have many adverse side effects and be highly addictive.

Natural painkillers may also have applications in treating acute pain, such as post-operative pain. Some natural painkillers, such as ginger and turmeric, have been shown to have anti-inflammatory properties and may help reduce pain and swelling after surgery. Others, such as arnica and St. John's wort, have analgesic properties and help reduce pain associated with injuries.

In addition to their pain-relieving properties, natural painkillers may also have other clinical applications. For example, some natural painkillers have been shown to have anti-anxiety and antidepressant effects, which may help treat anxiety and depression. Others may have anti-inflammatory or antioxidant properties, helpful in treating inflammatory conditions or as a general health supplement.

However, it is essential to note that natural painkillers are not without risks. Like any medication, they can have side effects and interact with other medicines. In addition, some natural painkillers, such as comfrey and kava, have been associated with liver toxicity and should be used cautiously or avoided altogether. Therefore, it is also vital to ensure that natural painkillers are obtained from a reputable source and used in the appropriate dosage.

CHAPTER 8

Chemical composition

Salicin

Salicin is a natural plant compound that belongs to the class of organic compounds known as glycosides. It is found in several plant species, including willow trees (Salix spp.), poplar trees (Populus spp.), and meadowsweet (Filipendula ulmaria). Salicin has a molecular formula of $C_{13}H_{18}O_7$ and a molecular weight of 286.28 g/mol.

The chemical structure of Salicin consists of a glucose molecule attached to a phenylpropanoid moiety, which in turn is linked to a salicylic acid molecule. The salicylic acid component is responsible for the pharmacological activity of Salicin, as it can be converted into salicylic acid in the body. Salicin is metabolised in the liver and converted into salicylic acid by esterases.

Studies have shown that Salicin possesses anti-inflammatory, analgesic, and antipyretic properties. Salicylic acid inhibits the production of prostaglandins in the body, which are involved in the inflammatory response. This action accounts for the ability of Salicin to reduce pain and inflammation. Salicin also inhibits the activity of cyclooxygenase enzymes, which are involved in synthesising prostaglandins.

Recent studies have explored the potential health benefits of Salicin for humans. For example, research has suggested that Salicin may have anticancer properties, as it has been shown to inhibit the growth of several cancer cells. In addition, Salicin has also been investigated for its potential as a treatment for osteoarthritis, as it has been shown to reduce pain and improve joint function in some studies.

In addition, Salicin has been shown to benefit cardiovascular health. It has been shown to reduce the risk of heart disease by lowering blood clotting and improving blood vessel function. Salicin may also have a role in preventing type 2 diabetes, as it has been shown to improve insulin sensitivity and glucose tolerance in some studies.

Salicin is a natural plant compound with many potential health benefits. Its chemical structure consists of a glucose molecule attached to a phenylpropanoid moiety and a salicylic acid molecule. Studies have shown that Salicin possesses anti-inflammatory, analgesic, and antipyretic properties and may have the potential as a treatment for cancer, osteoarthritis, and cardiovascular disease.

Interesting Facts:

Salicin is one of the oldest pain relievers in history. It's believed that Hippocrates, often called the "Father of Medicine," advised patients to chew on willow bark to reduce fever and inflammation.

The bark of the willow tree, which contains Salicin, was used as chew sticks by Native Americans to relieve pain and fever.

Bayer, a German pharmaceutical company, first synthesised aspirin (acetylsalicylic acid) from Salicin in the late 19th century, making it one of the first drugs ever made in a lab.

Salicin Through History: Willow bark as a natural remedy can be traced back to the ancient Egyptians, who used it to treat inflammation. The Greek physician Hippocrates wrote about the medicinal properties of willow bark in the 5th century BC.

In the 18th century, Reverend Edward Stone of Chipping Norton, England, rediscovered the therapeutic uses of willow bark, ultimately leading to Salicin's discovery and isolation in the 19th century.

Salicin Use by Wise Women of the Past: In ancient and medieval times, "wise women," often the de facto healers of their communities, would have likely known about and used willow bark for its medicinal properties. Given its widespread availability and efficacy as a pain reliever and fever reducer, it would have been a valuable component of their herbal medicine repertoire. It was also used in various forms, such as teas and poultices, to treat multiple ailments, from headaches to stomach complaints.

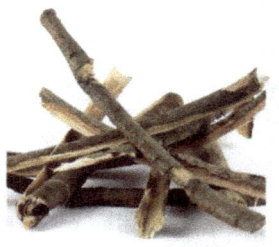 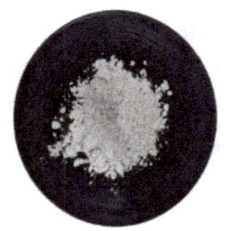

Hypericin and hyperforin

Hypericin and hyperforin are two natural compounds found in the plant species Hypericum perforatum, commonly known as St. John's Wort. St. John's Wort has been used for centuries as a traditional herbal medicine for various ailments, including depression, anxiety, and wound healing.

Hypericin is a naphthodianthrone derivative with a molecular formula of $C_{30}H_{16}O_8$ and a 504.45 g/mol molecular weight. Its chemical structure is a polycyclic aromatic hydrocarbon with a central oxygenated naphthalene system connected to a benzene ring. Hypericin is a red pigment that is highly phototoxic and can cause skin sensitivity to light.

Hyperforin is a prenylated phloroglucinol derivative with a molecular formula of C35H52O4 and a molecular weight of 536.8 g/mol. Its chemical structure consists of three isoprene units linked to a phloroglucinol moiety. Hyperforin is responsible for the antidepressant and anxiolytic properties of St. John's Wort.

Recent studies have investigated the potential health benefits of hypericin and hyperforin for humans. For example, hypericin has been shown to possess antiviral and antibacterial properties, which may help treat infectious diseases. It has also been shown to have anticancer effects, as it can induce apoptosis (programmed cell death) in cancer cells. In addition, hypericin is a potential treatment for neurological disorders, such as Alzheimer's disease and Parkinson's disease.

Hyperforin has been studied for its antidepressant and anxiolytic properties. It acts as a reuptake inhibitor of serotonin, dopamine, and norepinephrine, neurotransmitters in mood regulation. Hyperforin is effective in treating mild to moderate depression and has a similar efficacy to standard antidepressants. It has also been shown to have potential as a treatment for anxiety disorders.

It is essential to note that St. John's Wort can interact with several medications, including antidepressants, birth control pills, and blood thinners. Therefore, it is necessary to consult a healthcare professional before taking St. John's Wort or any other herbal supplement.

In conclusion, hypericin and hyperforin are two natural compounds in St. John's Wort with potential health benefits. Hypericin has antiviral, antibacterial, anticancer, and neuroprotective properties, while hyperforin has antidepressant and anxiolytic properties. However, caution should be exercised when using St. John's Wort due to its potential drug interactions.

Scientific Studies: Schempp CM et al. published a paper titled "Hyperforin acts as an anti-inflammatory agent in the Acutely Inflamed Skin" in the journal "Inflammation Research" (2003). They found that hyperforin inhibited certain types of inflammation in the skin.

A study by Savli E et al. titled "Investigation of anti-inflammatory activity of bergamot oil and hyperforin" in the journal "Natural Product Communications" (2012) explores the anti-inflammatory properties of hyperforin.

Another study by Novelle MG et al., "Effects of Hypericum perforatum extract in zebrafish: Evaluation of its behavioural and antioxidant effects", in the journal "Phytotherapy Research" (2013) discussed the antioxidant properties of St. John's wort, which can indirectly relate to anti-inflammatory effects.

Linalool

Linalool is a terpene alcohol commonly found in many plant species, including lavender, rosewood, and basil. It has a floral, spicy, and slightly woody scent and is widely used in the fragrance and flavouring industry. Linalool has a molecular formula of $C_{10}H_{18}O$ and a molecular weight of 154.25 g/mol.

Linalool is an important bioactive compound with a wide range of pharmacological properties, including antioxidant, anti-inflammatory, antinociceptive, anxiolytic, and sedative effects. These properties make linalool a potential therapeutic agent for various health conditions.

Recent studies have shown that linalool can modulate the immune response and reduce inflammation. For example, a study conducted in mice showed that linalool reduced inflammation in the lungs and airways, making it a potential treatment option for respiratory diseases such as asthma and chronic obstructive pulmonary disease (COPD).

Linalool has also been studied for its potential anxiolytic and sedative effects. A study conducted in humans showed that inhalation of linalool reduced anxiety levels and increased feelings of relaxation. Another study showed that linalool increased sleep time and decreased motor activity in mice, indicating its potential as a natural sleep aid.

In addition, linalool has been shown to have neuroprotective effects. A study conducted in rats showed that linalool protected against oxidative stress and improved cognitive function. This suggests that linalool may have potential as a therapeutic agent for treating neurodegenerative diseases such as Alzheimer's and Parkinson's.

Despite its potential health benefits, linalool can cause skin irritation and allergic reactions in some individuals. Therefore, it is crucial to use linalool-containing products cautiously and consult a healthcare professional before using them for medicinal purposes.

In conclusion, linalool is a terpene alcohol with various pharmacological properties, including antioxidant, anti-inflammatory, anxiolytic, and sedative effects. Recent studies have shown its potential as a therapeutic agent for treating respiratory diseases, anxiety, sleep disorders, and neurodegenerative diseases. However, caution should be exercised when using linalool-containing products due to the potential for skin irritation and allergic reactions.

Interesting fact: Linalool is found in over 200 species of plants, including mint, scented herbs, laurels, cinnamon, rosewood, and citrus fruits. It's most famously associated with lavender, contributing significantly to its signature scent.

Scientific Studies: "Effects of inhaled linalool in anxiety, social interaction and aggressive behaviour in mice" by Linck, VM, et al., published in "Phytomedicine" in 2010, investigated the anxiolytic effects of linalool.

A study titled "Anti-inflammatory effects of linalool in RAW 264.7 macrophages and lipopolysaccharide-induced lung injury model" by Peana, A.T., et al., published in "Journal of Surgical Research" in 2012, discusses linalool's potential anti-inflammatory properties.

In 2002, a study named "In vitro antimicrobial activity of essential oils from aromatic plants against selected food-borne pathogens" by Burt, S., published in "The Journal of Applied Microbiology", explored linalool's antimicrobial effects.

Neuroprotective Effects: A 2016 study by Sabogal-Guáqueta, A.M. et al., titled "The flavonoid quercetin ameliorates Alzheimer's disease pathology and protects cognitive and emotional function in aged triple transgenic Alzheimer's disease model mice" published in "Neuropharmacology" discusses the neuroprotective effects of linalool.

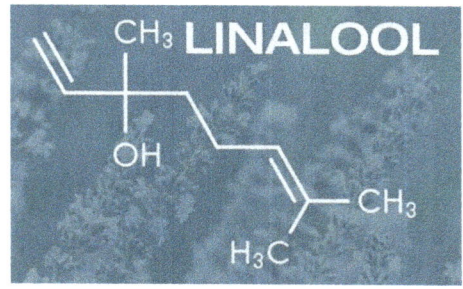

Betulinic acid, lupeol, and betulin

Betulinic acid, lupeol, and betulin are three triterpenoids in many plants, including birch trees and medicinal herbs. These compounds have gained attention recently due to their potential health benefits and therapeutic properties.

Betulinic acid has a molecular formula of $C_{30}H_{48}O_3$ and a molecular weight of 456.7 g/mol. It is a natural derivative of betulin found in the bark of the white birch tree. Betulinic acid has been shown to possess a wide range of biological activities, including antitumour, anti-inflammatory, antiviral, and antimalarial effects.

In addition, studies have demonstrated that betulinic acid can induce apoptosis (programmed cell death) in cancer cells and inhibit the growth of various cancer types, including melanoma, breast cancer, and prostate cancer.

Lupeol has a molecular formula of C30H50O and a molecular weight of 426.7 g/mol. It is a natural triterpenoid found in many plants, including mangoes, grapes, and medicinal herbs. Lupeol has been shown to possess a wide range of biological activities, including anti-inflammatory, antioxidant, antitumour, and antiviral effects. In addition, studies have shown that lupeol can inhibit the growth of various cancer types, including the colon, breast, and liver. It has also been shown to have the potential as a therapeutic agent for treating skin diseases, such as psoriasis and atopic dermatitis.

Betulin has a molecular formula of C30H50O2 and a molecular weight of 442.7 g/mol. It is a natural triterpenoid found in the bark of birch trees and other plants. Betulin has been shown to possess a wide range of biological activities, including anti-inflammatory, antioxidant, and antitumour effects. In addition, studies have shown that betulin can inhibit the growth of various cancer types, including melanoma, lung cancer, and prostate cancer.

Betulin has also been shown to have the potential as a therapeutic agent for the treatment of liver diseases, such as non-alcoholic fatty liver disease (NAFLD).

Recent studies have focused on the potential health benefits of these triterpenoids, particularly their anticancer properties. In one study, betulinic acid was shown to inhibit the growth of ovarian cancer cells and sensitise them to chemotherapy drugs. In another study, lupeol was shown to inhibit the growth of breast cancer cells and enhance the effectiveness of chemotherapy drugs. Betulin has also been shown to inhibit the growth of prostate cancer cells and sensitise them to radiation therapy.

In addition to their anticancer properties, these triterpenoids have also been shown to possess other health benefits. For example, betulinic acid has been shown to have the potential as a therapeutic agent for the treatment of HIV due to its ability to inhibit the replication of the virus. In addition, Lupeol has been shown to have potential as a therapeutic agent for treating Alzheimer's disease due to its ability to protect against neuronal damage.

Betulinic acid, lupeol, and betulin are three triterpenoids with potential health benefits and therapeutic properties. These compounds have been shown to possess anticancer, anti-inflammatory, antioxidant, and antiviral effects.

Recent studies have focused on their potential as therapeutic agents for treating cancer, HIV, Alzheimer's disease, and other health conditions. However, further research is needed to fully understand their potential health benefits and develop them as effective therapeutic agents.

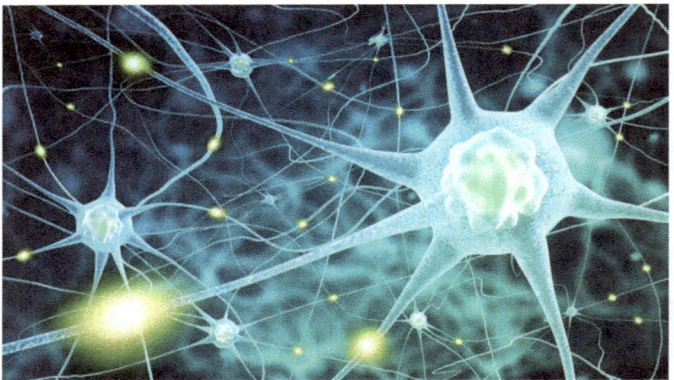

Neurotransmitters

"The creation of a thousand forests is in one acorn." - Ralph Waldo Emerson

Sesquiterpene lactones (STLs)

Sesquiterpene lactones (STLs) are a diverse natural product class found in many plants, particularly in the Asteraceae family. STLs are characterised by a lactone ring attached to a sesquiterpene (a compound containing three isoprene units) backbone. They are known for their diverse biological activities, including anti-inflammatory, antimicrobial, and anticancer effects.

STLs are structurally diverse and can be classified into subclasses based on the type of lactone ring and the substitution patterns of the sesquiterpene backbone. The most common types of lactone rings found in STLs are α-methylene-γ-lactone, α,β-unsaturated-γ-lactone, and γ-lactone. The sesquiterpene backbone can also be substituted with various functional groups, such as hydroxyl, methoxyl, and acetyl.

Recent studies have shown that STLs have potential health benefits for humans. For example, several studies have investigated the anticancer properties of STLs. One study found that the STL parthenolide inhibited the growth of pancreatic cancer cells and induced apoptosis.

Another study found that STL helenalin inhibited the growth of glioblastoma cells and induced cell death. Additionally, STLs have been shown to have anti-inflammatory effects, which may help treat inflammatory diseases such as rheumatoid arthritis and inflammatory bowel disease.

STLs also have antimicrobial properties, which have been investigated as a potential alternative to antibiotics. For example, one study found that the STL artemisinin, commonly used as an antimalarial drug, has antibacterial properties against several Gram-positive bacteria, including Staphylococcus aureus and Streptococcus pneumoniae.

Despite their potential health benefits, some STLs can also have toxic effects. For example, certain STLs have been shown to cause contact dermatitis, and others can cause liver toxicity. Therefore, caution should be taken when using STL-containing plants or products.

In conclusion, sesquiterpene lactones are a diverse class of natural products with potential health benefits for humans.

They have been shown to possess anti-inflammatory, antimicrobial, and anticancer properties. However, some STLs can also have toxic effects, and further research is needed to understand their potential health benefits and risks fully.

Lawsone

Lawsone, also known as hennotannic acid, is a natural organic compound found in the leaves of the henna plant (Lawsonia inermis) and the Jewelweed plant. It is a reddish-orange dye molecule used for centuries to colour hair, skin, and textiles in various cultures worldwide.

The chemical structure of Lawsone consists of a benzene ring with two hydroxyl groups (OH) and one ketone group (C=O) attached to it. It is a member of the naphthoquinone family of compounds known for their antioxidant and anti-inflammatory properties.

Recent studies have investigated Lawsone's potential health benefits, mainly its antioxidant and anti-inflammatory effects. One study found that Lawsone had potent antioxidant activity, as it could scavenge free radicals and protect against oxidative stress-induced damage in human liver cells. Another study found that Lawsone had anti-inflammatory effects, as it reduced the production of inflammatory cytokines in immune cells.

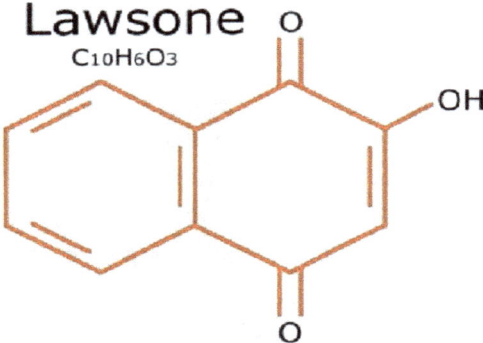

Lawsone $C_{10}H_6O_3$

2-Hydroxy-1,4-Naphthoquinone

Additionally, Lawsone has been investigated for its potential anticancer properties. One study found that Lawsone inhibited growth and induced apoptosis (programmed cell death) in human breast cancer cells. Another study found that Lawsone inhibited the growth and migration of human prostate cancer cells.

Lawsone has also been investigated for its potential use in wound healing. One study found that topical application of Lawsone increased the rate of wound closure and reduced inflammation in mice with excisional skin wounds. Another study found that Lawsone accelerated the healing of oral ulcers in human patients with recurrent aphthous stomatitis.

In addition to its potential health benefits, Lawsone has been used as a natural hair dye and for body art in various cultures. However, caution should be taken when using henna-based products, as some individuals may experience allergic reactions or sensitisation to the compound.

In conclusion, Lawsone is a natural organic compound in the henna and Jewelweed plants. That has potential health benefits, including antioxidant, anti-inflammatory, and anticancer properties and possible use in wound healing. However, further research is needed to understand its mechanisms of action and potential risks fully.

Aescin

Aescin, also known as escin, is a natural mixture of triterpene saponins found in the seeds of the horse chestnut tree (Aesculus hippocastanum). It is a complex chemical compound with a molecular weight of approximately 1131 g/mol. It comprises several different saponin molecules, including aescin Ia, aescin Ib, aescin IIa, and aescin Iib.

Aescin has been studied extensively for its potential health benefits, particularly its anti-inflammatory and antioxidant properties. In addition, it has been shown to have various effects on the cardiovascular system, including reducing oedema, improving blood circulation, and reducing the risk of blood clots.

One study found that aescin inhibited the production of inflammatory cytokines and chemokines in human immune cells, suggesting that it may help treat inflammatory conditions such as arthritis and asthma. Another study found that aescin reduced the severity of acute lung injury in mice by inhibiting the production of inflammatory molecules.

Aescin has also been investigated for its potential use in treating chronic venous insufficiency, a condition characterised by poor blood flow in the veins of the legs. Several studies have shown that aescin can reduce leg swelling and improve blood circulation in individuals with this condition. For example, in one study, aescin was as effective as compression stockings for reducing leg swelling in individuals with chronic venous insufficiency.

In addition to its potential health benefits, aescin has been used in the cosmetic industry for its anti-inflammatory and anti-ageing properties. It is commonly found in creams and lotions designed to reduce puffiness and dark circles around the eyes. However, it is essential to note that aescin can have side effects, including stomach upset, nausea, and headache. It may also interact with certain medications, so it is essential to consult with a healthcare professional before taking Aescin.

In conclusion, aescin is a natural mixture of triterpene saponins found in the seeds of the horse chestnut tree that has potential health benefits, including anti-inflammatory and antioxidant properties, as well as possible use in treating chronic venous insufficiency. However, further research is needed to understand its mechanisms of action and potential risks fully.

Lactucarium

Lactucarium is a milky sap secreted by certain lettuce species (Lactuca spp.). It has been used historically for its sedative and analgesic properties and is often referred to as "lettuce opium" due to its similar effects to opium. The chemical composition of lactucarium is complex and includes lactucin, lactucopicrin, and other related lactones.

Lactucin is a sesquiterpene lactone found in lactucarium that has been shown to have sedative effects. It acts on the central nervous system by binding to GABA-A receptors, which are involved in the regulation of anxiety and sleep. In one study, lactucin significantly increased sleeping time in mice, suggesting its potential as a natural sleep aid.

Lactucopicrin is another significant component of lactucarium that has been shown to have analgesic properties. It has been found to inhibit the production of prostaglandins and leukotrienes, which are involved in the inflammatory response and pain perception. In one study, lactucopicrin significantly reduced pain in mice induced with inflammatory pain.

Lactucarium has also been investigated for its potential use in treating anxiety and depression. One study found that lactucarium had anxiolytic effects in mice, reducing anxiety-like behaviour and increasing levels of brain-derived neurotrophic factor (BDNF), a protein involved in the growth and survival of neurons. In another study, lactucarium was found to have antidepressant effects in rats, increasing levels of serotonin and noradrenaline in the brain. However, it is essential to note that lactucarium can have side effects, including nausea, vomiting, and dizziness. It may also interact with certain medications, so it is necessary to consult with a healthcare professional before using lactucarium supplements.

In conclusion, lactucarium is a milky sap secreted by certain lettuce species with potential sedative, analgesic, anxiolytic, and antidepressant effects. Its major components include lactucin and lactucopicrin, which have been shown to act on the central nervous system and inhibit the production of inflammatory molecules. However, further research is needed to understand its mechanisms of action and potential risks fully.

Phenol

Phenol, also known as carbolic acid, is a white crystalline compound with the molecular formula C_6H_5OH. It is an aromatic compound with a benzene ring attached to a hydroxyl group. While phenol is manufactured industrially and used in resins, plastics, and pharmaceuticals, it is also found naturally in certain plants. In natural medicine, phenolic compounds are noteworthy for their potential analgesic (pain-relieving) and other medicinal properties.

The chemical structure of phenol features a hydroxyl group (-OH) attached to a benzene ring. This configuration confers specific properties of the compound, including its ability to act as a weak acid and its reactivity with other compounds. Plants synthesise phenolic compounds to defend against pathogens, herbivores, and environmental stresses. These compounds play a vital role in the plant's ability to withstand multiple external pressures and can contribute to the plant's medicinal properties.

Some phenolic compounds found in plants have shown potential analgesic properties. They may work by various mechanisms, such as reducing inflammation or inhibiting the transmission of pain signals. The anti-inflammatory properties of phenolic compounds are fascinating, as inflammation is often associated with pain. By reducing inflammation, phenolic compounds may help to alleviate pain and discomfort.

Phenolic compounds also exhibit antioxidant properties. They can neutralise free radicals in the body, reducing oxidative stress and potentially preventing various health issues, including chronic diseases and conditions associated with inflammation and oxidative damage.

The antimicrobial properties of phenolic compounds contribute to their potential use in natural medicine. By inhibiting the growth of bacteria, fungi, and other pathogens, phenolic compounds may help to prevent or treat infections. Eugenol, a phenolic compound found in Wood Avens, exhibits analgesic and anti-inflammatory properties. While phenol and phenolic compounds found in plants have shown potential as natural analgesics and have other medicinal properties, researchers must conduct more comprehensive, high-quality clinical trials to investigate their safety and effectiveness further.

Natural does not always mean safe, and it's essential to consider the dosage, side effects, and potential interactions with other medications before using any natural remedy for pain relief or other health issues.

Glucosides

Glucosides do not have a single molecular structure because they are a large class of compounds. A glucoside generally consists of a glucose molecule bonded to another functional group, called an aglycone, through a glycosidic linkage. The aglycone can be different molecules, so the exact structure of a glucoside depends on what that aglycone is.

The glucose part of a glucoside is a six-carbon (hexose) sugar molecule. It is typically represented in a ring form, where five carbons and one oxygen form the ring, and the remaining carbon is attached as a side group. The aglycone part of a glucoside can be any of various molecules, including other sugars, phenolic compounds, terpenes, or many others.

The glycosidic linkage is a covalent bond that attaches the glucose molecule to the aglycone. It is formed by a reaction between a hydroxyl group (-OH) on the glucose molecule and a hydroxyl group on the aglycone, releasing a water molecule.

Glucosides are a diverse group of compounds found in plants, consisting of a glucose molecule bonded to another functional group, often a non-sugar molecule. This chemical structure allows glucosides to partake in various biological activities, including potential roles in natural medicine and pain relief.

Glucosides have a basic chemical structure that includes a glucose (or sugar) molecule and another molecule, often a non-carbohydrate structure, called the aglycone. The bond between the glucose and aglycone is a glycosidic linkage. The aglycone portion can be a wide range of compounds, contributing to the diversity of glucosides and their various biological activities.

In plants, glucosides perform various functions, including acting as a reservoir for secondary metabolites, which play a role in the plant's defence mechanism against pests and pathogens. The stored compounds can be released by enzymatic hydrolysis, which cleaves the glycosidic bond, releasing the aglycone, which often has bioactive properties.

Some glucosides found in plants may have analgesic (pain-relieving) properties. The released aglycone, upon hydrolysis, may interact with various biological targets in the human body to exert a pain-relieving effect.

Glucosides can also have anti-inflammatory effects. The aglycone portion may modulate the activity of various enzymes and pathways involved in the inflammatory response, potentially relieving inflammation-related pain and discomfort.

The aglycone portion of glucosides can also exhibit antioxidant properties, neutralising harmful free radicals in the body. This action can help prevent oxidative stress, inflammation, and related health issues. Other health benefits of glucosides include antimicrobial, antiviral, and anticancer activities.

Glucosides found in plants have the potential to contribute to natural medicine, including acting as analgesics and offering other health benefits. However, just like all-natural compounds, it is crucial to approach their use cautiously.

Comprehensive research, including clinical trials, is essential to ascertain their safety, efficacy, optimal dosage, and potential interactions with other medications. Proper consultation with healthcare professionals is always recommended before incorporating any new substance into a health regimen.

Keytones

Ketones are a group of organic compounds characterised by a carbonyl group (C=O) bonded to two alkyl or aryl groups. They are widespread and are found in various plants, where they play significant roles in plant metabolism and defence. Beyond this, some plant ketones have potential applications in natural medicine, including pain relievers or analgesics.

Ketones have a simple chemical structure: a carbonyl group (C=O) is bonded to two other carbon atoms. This structure is represented as RC (=O)R', where R and R' are alkyl or aryl groups. The specific properties of a ketone depend on these groups.

In plants, ketones participate in various biological processes, including growth, respiration, and the synthesis of complex molecules. Some plant ketones also act as signalling molecules or defence compounds that protect plants against pests and pathogens.

Particular ketones found in plants exhibit potential analgesic properties, possibly acting on the nervous system to inhibit the transmission of pain signals. Some may interact with specific receptors or enzymes in the pain pathway, providing a basis for developing new pain relief medications.

Some plant-derived ketones may have anti-inflammatory effects, reducing inflammation by modulating immune responses or inhibiting enzymes involved in the inflammatory process. This anti-inflammatory activity can contribute to their analgesic products, as inflammation often accompanies pain.

Ketones can have other health benefits, such as antioxidant, antimicrobial, and antiviral activities. By reducing oxidative stress and inhibiting pathogen growth, ketones contribute to overall health and well-being.

Ketones found naturally in various plants hold promise for natural medicine, including potential use as analgesics. Their diverse structures and biological activities contribute to their varied medicinal properties.

"A weed is but an unloved flower." - Ella Wheeler Wilcox

CHAPTER 9

Optimising Natural Pain Relief: Lifestyle Integration, Proper Handling, and Safe Use

Integrating Natural Painkillers into Your Lifestyle

Using natural painkillers from native U.K. trees, plants, and fungi can be a great way to manage pain while avoiding the potential side effects of synthetic drugs. However, it is essential to remember that natural remedies are not a substitute for professional medical advice and treatment.

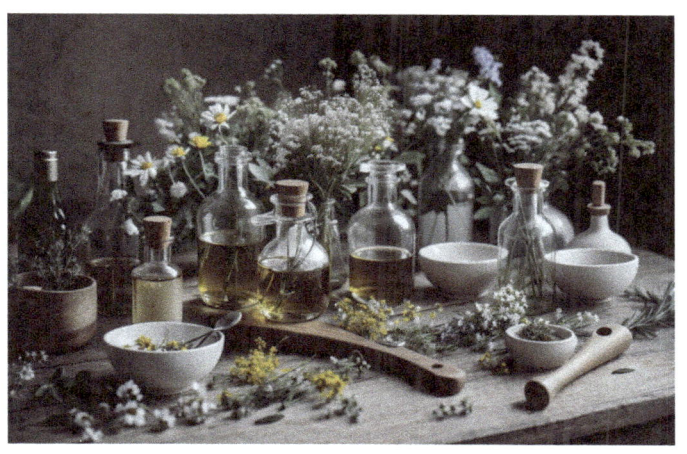

Here are some ways to integrate natural painkillers into your lifestyle:

Consult with a healthcare professional: If you are experiencing chronic pain or other serious health issues, it is crucial to seek professional medical advice. Discuss using natural painkillers with your healthcare provider to ensure they are safe and appropriate for your condition.

Learn about different remedies: Educate yourself on the natural painkillers available and their properties. This will help you make informed decisions about which treatments are best suited to your individual needs.

Harvest and prepare remedies properly: Follow proper harvesting and preparation methods to ensure the effectiveness and safety of natural remedies. This may include drying, grinding, or extracting the active compounds from the plant or fungi.

Start with small doses: When using natural remedies, start with a small amount and gradually increase it over time. This will help you gauge your body's response to the treatment and avoid potential adverse effects.

Maintain a healthy lifestyle: Incorporate natural painkillers into a healthy lifestyle that includes regular exercise, a balanced diet, and stress reduction techniques. This will help to manage pain and promote overall wellness.

Be aware of potential interactions: Natural painkillers may interact with other medications or supplements you take. Be sure to inform your healthcare provider of any remedies you are using to avoid potentially harmful interactions.

Keep records: Record the natural painkillers you use, the dosages, and any side effects or changes in your pain levels. This will help you track the effectiveness of the remedies and make adjustments as needed.

By integrating natural painkillers into your lifestyle safely and responsibly, you can effectively manage pain while promoting overall health and wellness.

Importance of Preparation, Storage, and

Dosage of Natural Remedies

While natural remedies can effectively treat pain and other ailments, it is essential to prepare, store, and dose them correctly to ensure their safety and efficacy.

Preparation: Many natural remedies require specific preparation methods to extract their active compounds. For example, teas and infusions are often used to remove active compounds from plants, while tinctures are used to extract compounds from roots and bark.

Therefore, it is crucial to follow the correct preparation method to obtain the desired concentration of active compounds and ensure that the remedy is effective.

Storage: To maintain potency, natural remedies should be stored in a cool, dry place. Exposure to light, heat, and moisture can degrade the active compounds in the remedy, rendering it ineffective. Therefore, storing natural remedies in airtight containers is essential to prevent contamination and preserve freshness.

Dosage: Natural remedies should be carefully dosed to avoid side effects and ensure their safety. Dosage can vary depending on the type of remedy, the individual's weight and age, and the severity of the condition being treated.

Awareness of potential interactions between natural remedies and other medications or health conditions is also essential. For example, some natural remedies may interact with blood-thinning drugs or cause allergic reactions in individuals with specific allergies.

In addition, it is vital to obtain natural remedies from a reputable source. Many natural remedies are available online or in health food stores, but not all products are of the same quality or purity. Therefore, it is essential to research the product and the company before purchasing it to ensure it is safe and effective.

In conclusion, preparation, storage, and dosage are crucial when using natural remedies for pain and other ailments. Therefore, following the correct preparation method is essential, as storing remedies in the proper conditions and dosing them carefully to ensure their safety and efficacy. It is also necessary to be aware of potential interactions and to obtain remedies from a reputable source.

Precautions and Disclaimers for Using Natural Remedies

While natural remedies can effectively treat pain and other ailments, exercising caution and taking certain precautions when using them is essential.

Here are some important considerations to keep in mind

Please consult with a healthcare practitioner: Before starting any natural remedy regimen, it is essential to consult with a qualified healthcare practitioner. They can advise on the appropriate remedy for your condition and guide dosing and potential side effects. In addition, it is imperative to consult a healthcare practitioner if you are pregnant, nursing, taking medication, or have a pre-existing health condition.

Please do not use it as a substitute for medical treatment: Natural remedies should never be used as a substitute for medical treatment. While they can effectively manage pain and other symptoms, they should always be used in conjunction with medical treatment, not instead.

Use caution: Natural remedies can have side effects or interact with other medications or health conditions. Therefore, starting with a low dose and monitoring for adverse effects is essential. If you experience adverse effects, discontinue use immediately and consult a healthcare practitioner.

Be aware of potential allergens: Some natural remedies, such as herbs or fungi, can cause allergic reactions in specific individuals. Therefore, it is essential to be mindful of any allergies and carefully read the label of any natural remedy you plan to use.

Quality and purity: Not all natural remedies are created equal. Researching the company and the product before purchasing is vital to ensure that it is of high quality and purity. Look for organic products that have undergone third-party testing for purity and potency.

Limitations of Natural Painkillers

While natural painkillers can be effective for many types of pain, they may not be appropriate for all kinds of pain or all individuals. Therefore, it is essential to understand the limitations of natural painkillers before using them. For example, natural painkillers may not be effective for severe or chronic pain and may not be appropriate for individuals with certain medical conditions or who are taking certain medications.

Risks and Side Effects: Natural painkillers can carry risks and side effects like any medication or treatment. For example, some natural painkillers may cause side effects such as dizziness, nausea, or allergic reactions. Additionally, some natural painkillers can interact with other medications, which can cause adverse effects.

Conclusion: In conclusion, natural painkillers can be a safe and effective option for many types of pain. Still, awareness of their limitations, potential risks, and side effects are essential. Therefore, before using natural painkillers, it is necessary to do your research, and make an informed decision about whether they are appropriate for you.

"Mushrooms are miniature pharmaceutical factories, and of the thousands of mushroom species in nature, our ancestors and modern scientists have identified several dozen that have a unique combination of talents that improve our health." - Paul Stamets

CHAPTER 10

From Field to Medicine Cabinet:

Native Species and Their Therapeutic

Preparation

Species

Willow Bark

Willow bark has been used for centuries as a natural painkiller and is still commonly used today. It is derived from the bark of several species of the willow tree, including white willow, black willow, and crack willow. The bark contains a compound called salicin, similar in structure to aspirin and effectively reduces pain and inflammation.

To prepare willow bark, you can brew it as a tea or use it in a tincture. To make tea, steep 1-2 teaspoons of dried willow bark in hot water for 10-15 minutes. To make a tincture, soak the bark in alcohol for several weeks, then strain and store it in a dark bottle.

Dosage recommendations vary depending on the preparation and the individual, so starting with a small amount is crucial, and gradually increasing the dosage as needed. Please note that willow bark should not be taken by individuals who are allergic to aspirin or have a bleeding disorder.

Fun Fact:

Willow bark was one of the first painkillers used by ancient civilisations, including the Egyptians and the Greeks. Hippocrates, the father of medicine, recommended willow bark for pain relief as early as the 5th Century BCE.

Quote: "The willow is my favourite tree. I grew up near one. It's the most flexible tree in nature, and nothing can break it – no wind, no elements, it can bend and withstand anything." - Pink

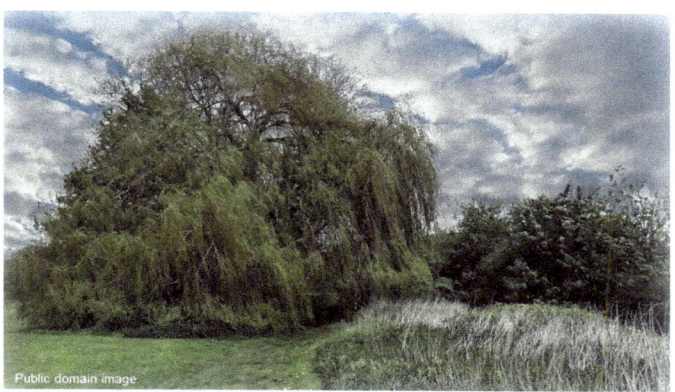

Willow Tree

Oh, the willow tree of the U.K. land

Oh, willow of British earth so fine,
Your boughs gracefully curve, almost divine,
Across the dales, beside babbling brooks,
You calm the heart with just a look.

Emerald fronds, they softly cascade,
Whispering secrets when winds persuade,
Elegance is captured in every pose,
Elevating spirits, easing woes.

When spring graces, tender sprouts emerge,
Signalling nature's invigorating surge,
With every budding, a melodic tune rings,
Celebrating life as the verdant realm sings.

In the sun-drenched days of summertime's dance,
You offer a haven, a tranquil expanse,
Under your shade, souls find their peace,
Watching the world, its bustle ceases.

Autumn adorns you in radiant gold,
A prelude to tales of winter, untold,
Leaves pirouetting in a crisp air's kiss,
Foretelling of seasonal slumber and bliss.

Winter paints you in outlines so clear,
Against a canvas of chill, devoid of cheer,
Yet, nestled within, a silent vow grows,
Of rejuvenation and the warmth that follows.

Willow, iconic sentinel of Britain's terrain,
Nature's masterpiece, in sun or rain,
Through every season, you stand tall and cope,
Gifting us visions of perpetual hope.

Harvesting and Preparation

Willow bark can be harvested from the tree in the early spring or autumn when the bark is most pliable. The bark should be removed from branches less than 2 inches in diameter to avoid damaging the tree. The bark can be harvested by making a horizontal cut around the circumference of the branch and then making a vertical cut down the length of the branch. The bark can then be peeled off in sections.

The bark should be dried in a well-ventilated area, away from direct sunlight, until it is crispy and brittle. Once dry, the bark can be ground into a fine powder using a mortar, pestle, or coffee grinder. It can then be stored in an airtight container in a cool, dark place for up to a year.

Dosage: The appropriate dosage of willow bark can vary depending on the individual and the treated condition. Therefore, starting with a low dose and gradually increasing it as needed is recommended.

A typical dosage is 240 mg of salicin daily, equivalent to 1-2 teaspoons of dried willow bark powder.

Benefits: Willow bark has effectively reduced pain and inflammation, particularly in osteoarthritis, rheumatoid arthritis, and lower back pain. For example, a systematic review of 15 clinical trials found that willow bark extract effectively reduced pain and improved physical function in individuals with osteoarthritis. Another study found that willow bark extract was as effective as a prescription nonsteroidal anti-inflammatory drug (NSAID) in reducing pain and inflammation in individuals with rheumatoid arthritis.

In addition to its pain-relieving properties, willow bark has also been shown to have antipyretic (fever-reducing) and anti-platelet (blood-thinning) effects. These properties can be beneficial in treating fevers, headaches, and cardiovascular disease.

Safety and Side Effects: Willow bark is generally considered safe when used as directed. However, it can have side effects, mainly when used in high doses or for extended periods. Side effects can include stomach upset, nausea, vomiting, and allergic reactions. It should not be used by individuals allergic to aspirin or other NSAIDs.

Conclusion: Willow bark is a natural pain reliever that has been used for centuries. It is derived from the bark of several species of the willow tree and contains salicin, a natural form of aspirin. Willow bark has effectively reduced pain and inflammation, particularly in osteoarthritis, rheumatoid arthritis, and lower back pain. It also has antipyretic and anti-platelet effects that can be beneficial in treating fevers, headaches, and cardiovascular disease. However, it is vital to use willow bark with caution and under the guidance of a healthcare practitioner, particularly if you have a pre-existing health condition or are taking medication.

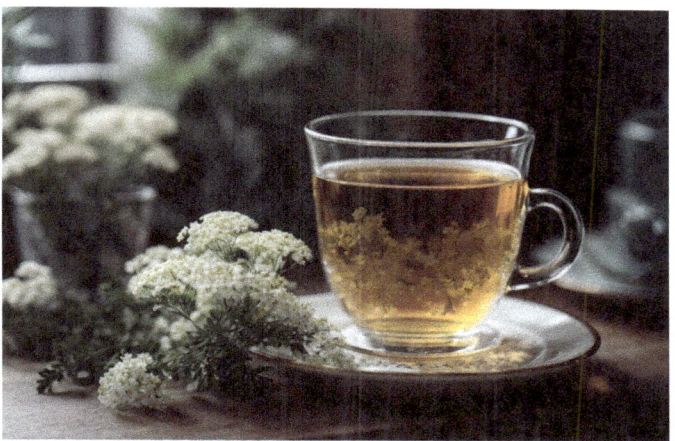

Meadowsweet

Meadowsweet (Filipendula ulmaria) is a perennial herb from the rose family (Rosaceae). It grows in damp meadows, ditches, and hedgerows throughout the U.K. and other parts of Europe and Asia. Meadowsweet has a long history of medicinal use and has been traditionally used to treat pain, fever, and digestive disorders.

Harvesting: Meadowsweet flowers are usually harvested in July and August when they are in full bloom. The flowers should be picked early in the day after the dew has evaporated but before the sun is too hot. The leaves can be harvested at any time during the growing season, but they are most potent when picked in early summer. Therefore, gathering only from areas not treated with herbicides or pesticides is vital.

Preparation: The flowers and leaves of meadowsweet can be used to make tea, tincture, or infused oil. To make tea, steep one teaspoon of dried meadowsweet flowers or leaves in a cup of hot water for 10-15 minutes. The tea can be sweetened with honey or stevia and consumed thrice daily.

To make a tincture, the flowers and leaves are soaked in alcohol for several weeks. The resulting tincture can be taken orally in small doses, usually 1-2 teaspoons, up to three times a day.

For several weeks, the infused oil can be made by soaking the flowers or leaves in a carrier oil such as olive or coconut oil. Then, the oil can be applied topically to the affected area for pain relief.

Dosage: The recommended dosage for meadowsweet varies depending on the preparation method. As tea, up to three cups per day can be consumed. As a tincture, 1-2 teaspoons can be taken up to three times daily. As a topical oil, a small amount can be applied to the affected area as needed.

Benefits: Meadowsweet has been found to contain salicylates, similar to aspirin and can help reduce pain and inflammation. Also, meadowsweet includes tannins, which can help soothe irritated tissue and reduce fever. It has also been traditionally used to relieve digestive disorders such as acid reflux and gastritis.

Studies

Several studies have been conducted on the pain-relieving effects of meadowsweet. For example, researchers in a study published in Phytomedicine Journal found that meadowsweet extracts effectively reduced pain in patients with knee osteoarthritis. Another study published in the Journal of Ethnopharmacology found that meadowsweet extract had anti-inflammatory effects in mice with induced paw oedema.

Overall, meadowsweet is a natural pain reliever used for centuries for its medicinal properties. However, as with any herbal remedy, it is essential to consult a healthcare professional before use, especially if you take any medications or have any underlying medical conditions.

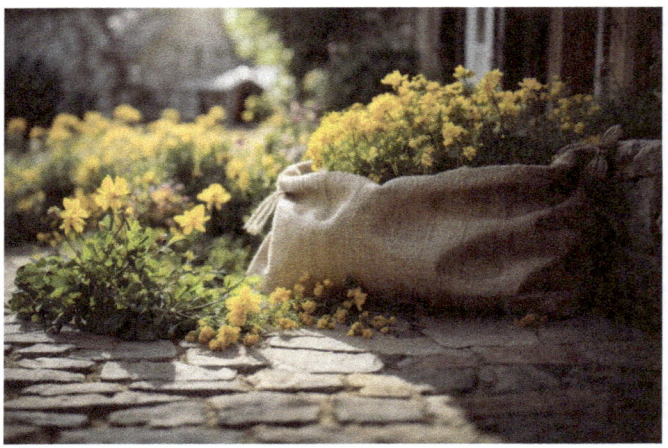

St. John's Wort

St. John's Wort

St. John's Wort, also known as Hypericum perforatum, is a perennial plant native to Europe but can also be found in North America, Asia, and Australia. It has been traditionally used as a natural remedy for various conditions, including depression, anxiety, nerve pain, and inflammation.

Harvesting: St. John's Wort blooms in late June or early July. The plant's flowering tops are the most commonly used medicinal parts. Harvesting the flowering tops on a sunny day when the plant is dry is best. The flowers should be picked when fully open, and the buds are just starting to open. Handling the plant with care is essential, as it can cause skin irritation and sensitivity to sunlight.

Preparation and Storage: Once harvested, the flowering tops can be dried later. They should be dried in a warm, dry place, out of direct sunlight. Once dried, they can be stored in an airtight container in a cool, dry place for up to a year.

Dosage and Benefits: St. John's Wort can be prepared in a tea, tincture, or capsule form. The recommended dosage for St. John's Wort is typically 300-900mg per day. It is essential to follow the recommended dosage as higher doses can cause side effects such as nausea, dry mouth, and dizziness.

St. John's Wort contains several compounds, including hypericin and hyperforin, which are believed to be responsible for their therapeutic effects.

It is commonly used as a natural remedy for mild to moderate depression, as several studies have shown it is effective in improving symptoms. In addition, St. John's Wort may also have anti-inflammatory and antiviral properties, making it a potential treatment for conditions such as herpes and HIV.

It is important to note that St. John's Wort can interact with certain medications, including antidepressants, birth control pills, and blood thinners. Therefore, it should only be combined with these medications by consulting a healthcare professional. St. John's Wort should also not be used during pregnancy or breastfeeding.

Conclusion: St. John's Wort is a natural remedy used for centuries to treat various conditions. However, following proper harvesting, preparation, and storage techniques is essential to ensure its safety and effectiveness. Therefore, while it may have therapeutic benefits, it should be used with caution and under the guidance of a healthcare professional, especially when combined with other medications.

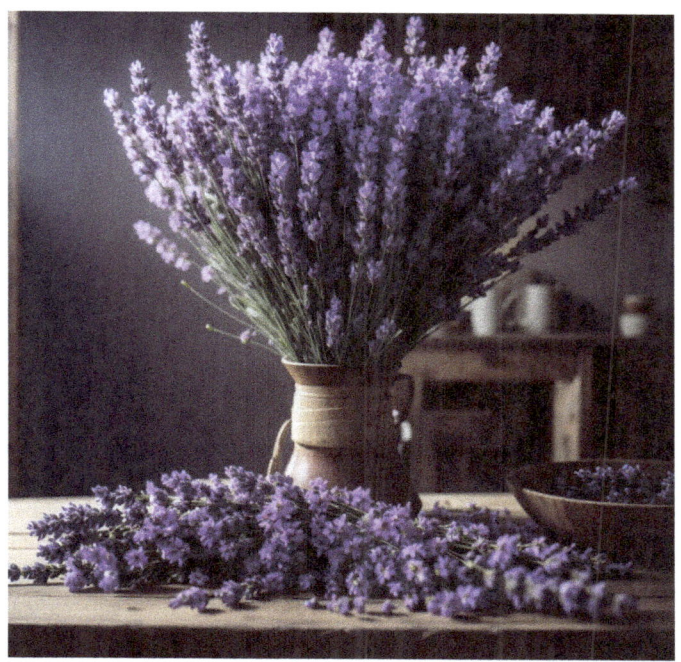

Lavender flowers

Lavender Oil

Lavender oil is extracted from the flowers of the lavender plant. The oil is often used in aromatherapy to promote relaxation and improve sleep quality. It is also used as a natural remedy for headaches and other types of pain.

Benefits and Mechanisms of Action: Lavender and lavender oil have been shown to have various health benefits, including pain relief. In addition, lavender oil may work by inhibiting the transmission of pain signals in the brain and spinal cord. In addition to its painkilling effects, lavender oil has been shown to have anti-inflammatory, antifungal, and antibacterial properties. It has also been used to treat anxiety, depression, and insomnia.

Dosage and Precautions: Lavender oil can be used in various ways, including aromatherapy, massage, and topical application. When using lavender oil topically, it is essential to dilute it with a carrier oil such as coconut or jojoba oil to avoid skin irritation.

It is generally safe to use lavender and lavender oil, but it is important to note that some people may be allergic to them. If you experience any adverse effects, discontinue use and consult a healthcare professional.

Conclusion: Lavender and lavender oil are natural remedies that may help alleviate pain and promote relaxation. While more research is needed to fully understand the mechanisms of action and potential side effects, these natural remedies have been used for centuries and are generally considered safe. Lavender is a widely used herb for its therapeutic benefits and calming and relaxing effects. However, the chemical composition of lavender varies depending on the species, subspecies, and the part of the plant used. Lavender contains various compounds, such as linalool, linalyl acetate, camphor, terpinen-4-ol, and lavandulol, contributing to its aromatic and medicinal properties.

Linalool is the major component of lavender essential oil, accounting for approximately 30-50% of the oil. It is known for its sedative and anxiolytic effects and has been shown to reduce anxiety in clinical studies. Linalyl acetate is another significant component of lavender oil, accounting for approximately 20-35% of the oil. It has been shown to have anxiolytic effects and can help improve sleep quality.

Camphor is a minor component of lavender oil, accounting for less than 1%, but it has been shown to have analgesic effects and is often used in topical pain relievers. Terpinen-4-ol is another minor component of lavender oil shown to have antifungal and antibacterial properties.

Lavender has been studied for its therapeutic effects on various conditions, including anxiety, insomnia, and pain. For example, a study published in the Journal of Alternative and Complementary Medicine found that inhaling lavender essential oil reduced anxiety in patients undergoing dental treatment. Another study published in Evidence-Based Complementary and Alternative Medicine found that lavender aromatherapy improved sleep quality in post-partum women.

A systematic review published in the journal Pain Medicine found that lavender essential oil effectively reduced pain and anxiety in patients undergoing medical procedures. In addition, a study published in the Phytotherapy Research Journal found that topical lavender oil reduced pain and inflammation in knee osteoarthritis patients.

Scientific studies suggest lavender and oil have therapeutic benefits, particularly in anxiety, sleep, and pain relief. However, more research is needed to understand further the mechanisms of action and potential side effects of using lavender and lavender oil as natural painkillers.

Chanterelle Mushroom

Chanterelle mushrooms, also known as Cantharellus cibarius, are a type of wild mushroom found in forests throughout the U.K. and other parts of Europe. They are known for their fruity aroma and delicate flavour and are often used in culinary dishes. However, they also have potential health benefits and have been used for centuries in traditional medicine.

Harvesting: Chanterelle mushrooms typically grow in the wild and can be found in deciduous and coniferous forests from midsummer through autumn. They are often found growing in clusters around the bases of trees or in damp, shaded areas. When harvesting, it is crucial to identify the mushroom to avoid picking poisonous lookalikes correctly. In addition, Chanterelle mushrooms should be carefully cut at the base of the stem to avoid damaging the surrounding area.

Preparation and Storage: After harvesting, Chanterelle mushrooms should be cleaned by gently brushing off any dirt or debris with a soft brush. They should not be washed or soaked in water, as this can cause them to become waterlogged and lose their delicate flavour.

Chanterelle mushrooms can be cooked immediately or stored in a paper bag in the refrigerator for up to five days.

Dosage and Benefits: Chanterelle mushrooms contain several bioactive compounds, including polysaccharides and beta-glucans, which have been shown to have potential health benefits. They may have anti-inflammatory and antioxidant properties, making them helpful in treating arthritis and cancer.

While there is limited research on the health benefits of Chanterelle mushrooms, a 2018 review of the potential health benefits of wild mushrooms found that they may have anti-inflammatory and immunomodulatory effects and could help treat conditions such as cancer, diabetes, and cardiovascular disease.

In terms of dosage, Chanterelle mushrooms can be consumed in moderation as part of a balanced diet. However, it is vital to correctly identify and cook them to avoid any potential adverse effects.

Conclusion

Chanterelle mushrooms are wild mushrooms found in forests throughout the U.K. and Europe. While they are primarily used in culinary dishes, they may also have potential health benefits due to their bioactive compounds. Proper harvesting, preparation, and cooking techniques should be followed to ensure the safety and enjoyment of these mushrooms. As with any natural remedy, it is essential to consult with a healthcare professional before use, especially if you have any underlying health conditions or are taking medications.

Interesting fact: Chanterelles contain just 17 calories per cup and provide a good source of vitamins and minerals, including vitamins D, A, E and C, several B vitamins, potassium, selenium, manganese, copper, iron and phosphorus. They are higher in vitamin D than commercially grown mushrooms and can contain between 60 to 100 per cent of your daily recommended intake per cup. Vitamin D is a significant anti-inflammatory and helps to maintain bone health. It is essential for people over 50, who need more vitamin D than younger people, and vegetarians and vegans, who have limited sources.

The compound Ergosterol, a provitamin form of vitamin D2, is found in high amounts in chanterelle mushrooms. When exposed to ultraviolet (UV) light, Ergosterol can convert to vitamin D2.

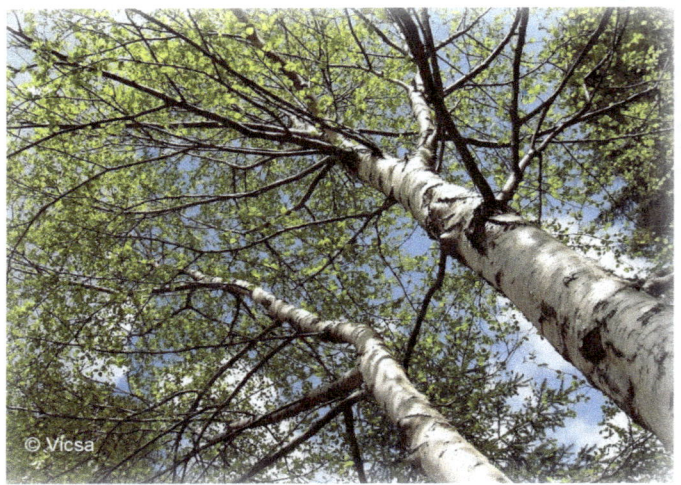

Birch Tree

Birch Bark - A Natural Painkiller

Birch bark is a well-known natural painkiller used by various cultures worldwide for centuries. The bark of the birch tree (Betula spp.) is rich in compounds such as salicylates, which have been found to have potent pain-relieving properties.

Chemical Composition: Birch bark comprises several chemical compounds, including betulinic acid, lupeol, betulin, and salicylates. Salicylates are the active compounds that provide the pain-relieving effects of birch bark. Salicylates are similar in structure to aspirin and work by inhibiting the production of prostaglandins, which are responsible for inflammation and pain in the body.

Mechanisms of Action: Birch bark's pain-relieving effects are due to salicylates, which have been found to have potent anti-inflammatory and analgesic effects. Salicylates work by inhibiting the production of prostaglandins, which are responsible for pain and inflammation in the body. Additionally, salicylates have been found to inhibit nitric oxide production, which plays a role in pain perception.

Clinical Applications: Birch bark has been used for centuries to treat various ailments, including pain, inflammation, and fever. For example, studies have found that birch bark extract can effectively reduce pain associated with osteoarthritis and rheumatoid arthritis. Additionally, birch bark has been found to have anti-inflammatory effects, making it helpful in treating conditions such as inflammatory bowel disease and asthma.

Harvesting, Preparation, and Storage: Birch bark can be harvested from mature birch trees in the late spring or early summer. The outer bark can be peeled away from the tree in long strips and then dried in a cool, dry place. Once dried, the bark can be ground into a powder or used to make a tea or tincture.

When preparing birch bark tea, the bark should be simmered in water for at least 10 minutes to release the active compounds. Then, the tea can be sweetened with honey or other natural sweeteners and consumed up to three times daily. Birch bark tincture can be prepared by steeping it in alcohol for several weeks before straining and using it.

Birch bark should be stored in a cool, dry place away from direct sunlight. It is crucial to use birch bark within six months of harvesting to ensure maximum potency.

Dosage: The recommended dosage of birch bark varies depending on the form of the remedy. Consuming up to three cups daily is advised when using birch bark tea. Birch bark tincture should be taken in drops, with the recommended dosage varying between 10-30 drops, up to three times daily.

Precautions and Disclaimers for Using Birch Bark: While birch bark is generally considered safe, some precautions should be considered before using it as a natural painkiller. Birch bark should not be used by individuals allergic to aspirin or salicylates, as it may cause an allergic reaction. Additionally, individuals taking blood-thinning medications should not use birch bark, as it may increase risk.

Birch, birch, the healing tree

Oh birch, enigmatic healer of woodlands,
Your whispers echo from age-old sands,
White canvas adorns you; in emerald, you dance,
Yet, many are blind to your therapeutic trance.

From you springs an elixir, both rich and deep,
Alleviating agonies, giving solace to those who weep,
Steeped with fervour in a cauldron's embrace,
Births a potion that sets our souls apace.

Ancients revered you; in manuscripts, they wrote,
A curative bark, their ailments it smote,
Yet, in this era, with time's endless drill,
You remedy afflictions, and you always will.

Verdant foliage, tales of vigour they narrate,
Holding cosmic codes, life's energy they propagate,
Brewed into nectar, harmonious and neat,
It rejuvenates sinews and gives tired feet a beat.

Mystical birch, nature's balm, so green,
In dire moments, your strength is seen,
Gratitude fills us for the gifts you assign,
And for the elation in our hearts, so divine.

Statistics from studies: In the 2008 study published in the Journal of Ethnopharmacology, the researchers found that the tea made from birch bark reduced pain and inflammation in rats. Specifically, they found that the tea reduced the number of writhes (a sign of pain) in the rats by 48% compared to a control group and reduced the levels of inflammatory markers in their blood.

In the 2012 study published in the same journal, the researchers found that the birch bark extract reduced the production of inflammatory molecules in human cells in vitro. Specifically, they found that the extract reduced the levels of two cytokines (TNF-α and IL-6) by up to 40%.

The 2017 study published in the Journal of Natural Products found that betulin could reduce pain in mice. Specifically, they discovered that betulin reduced the time spent licking and biting the injected paw (a sign of pain) by 42% compared to a control group.

It's worth noting that these statistics are based on animal and in vitro studies, and more research is needed to determine the safety and effectiveness of birch bark and betulin in humans.

Additionally, more than statistics is required to provide a complete picture of the effectiveness of a treatment, as other factors such as study design, sample size, and potential biases must also be considered.

"Look deep into nature, and then you will understand everything better." - Albert Einstein

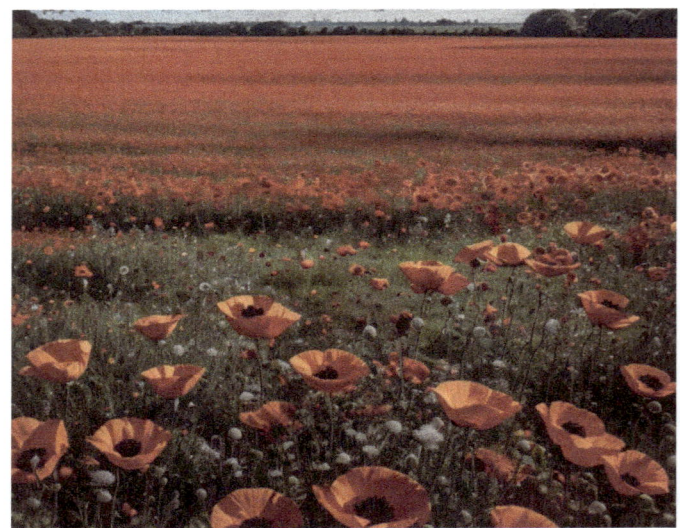

Poppies

Poppy

Poppy (Papaver somniferum) has been used for centuries for its pain-relieving properties. It is a flowering plant native to the eastern Mediterranean region but is now cultivated worldwide, including in the U.K. The opium poppy, the source of morphine, codeine, and other opioids, is a variety of P. somniferum.

Harvesting: Poppy plants are typically harvested when the seed pods are fully mature and the petals have fallen off. The latex that oozes out of the seed pods is collected and processed to obtain opium, which can be used directly or refined to obtain morphine, codeine, or other opioids.

Preparation and Storage: Poppy is available in various forms, including capsules, tablets, tinctures, and teas. Opium is also used in some traditional medicines, but it is a controlled substance in most countries and can only be obtained through a prescription. Poppy preparations should be stored in a cool, dry place away from direct sunlight.

Dosage: The appropriate dosage of poppy depends on several factors, including the individual's age, health status, and the specific product used. Therefore, following the manufacturer's instructions or a healthcare provider's recommendations when using poppy for pain relief is crucial.

Benefits: Poppy and its derivatives are potent pain relievers, especially for moderate to severe pain. They bind to specific brain and spinal cord receptors, reducing pain perception. Poppy also has sedative effects, which can help promote sleep and reduce anxiety. In addition to pain relief, the poppy has been used for its antitussive, antidiarrhoeal, and antispasmodic properties.

Studies: Several studies have investigated the analgesic properties of poppy and its derivatives. One study found that morphine, the main active ingredient in opium, is an effective pain reliever for cancer-related pain. Another study compared the efficacy of different doses of morphine and found that a low dose of morphine was just as effective as a higher dose for pain relief.

One study compared the effectiveness of codeine and ibuprofen for pain relief after oral surgery and found that codeine was more effective in reducing pain intensity and duration. However, codeine was associated with more adverse effects, including nausea and dizziness.

Another study investigated the use of poppy seed oil as a topical analgesic for pain relief in patients with osteoarthritis. The results showed that poppy seed oil effectively reduced pain and improved joint function.

Conclusion: Poppy and its derivatives are potent pain relievers with sedative effects. Therefore, they should only be used under medical supervision and caution due to the potential for addiction and adverse effects. Nevertheless, poppy remains an essential natural remedy for pain relief and is commonly used in modern medicine.

Some interesting facts about the poppy and its medicinal use:

- Poppy seeds are popular in baked goods, including bread and muffins. They contain small amounts of morphine and codeine, which can cause a positive result on a drug test if consumed in large quantities.

- Poppy seed oil is often used in skin and hair care products, as it is rich in fatty acids and has moisturising properties.

- Poppy flowers have been used in traditional medicine to treat insomnia, anxiety, and pain.

- In addition, tea made from flowers is said to have a calming effect on the body and mind.

- Poppy straw, the dried stems and leaves of the poppy plant, contains small amounts of morphine and codeine and has been used in traditional medicine to treat pain and coughs.

- Poppy extract is sometimes used in homoeopathic medicine to treat conditions such as anxiety, depression, and sleep disorders.

- Poppy tea, made by steeping poppy straw in hot water, is sometimes used as a natural painkiller. However, it can be dangerous if consumed in large quantities, as it can lead to respiratory depression and other serious side effects.

- Poppy has also been used in traditional medicine to treat skin conditions such as eczema and psoriasis and digestive issues such as constipation.

- When applied topically, poppy oil has been used in traditional medicine to treat earaches, toothaches, and headaches. It is said to have a numbing effect on the affected area.

- Poppy has been used in traditional medicine worldwide for centuries, and many of its uses have been validated by modern scientific research. However, it is essential to use poppy and its derivatives under the guidance of a healthcare professional, as they can be dangerous if misused.

"Someone's sitting in the shade today because someone planted a tree a long time ago." - Warren Buffett

Valerian Root

Valerian root (Valeriana officinalis) is a herbaceous perennial plant that belongs to the Valerianaceae family. It is native to Europe and parts of Asia but is now widely cultivated worldwide. Valerian root has been used as a medicinal herb for centuries due to its sedative and anxiolytic effects.

Harvesting Information: Valerian root is typically harvested in the autumn after the plant has completed its flowering stage. The roots are carefully dug out of the ground, washed, and dried. It is essential to handle the roots gently to avoid damaging them.

Preparation: Valerian root can be prepared in various ways, including as a tea, tincture, or capsule. To make valerian root tea, steep 1-2 teaspoons of dried valerian root in a cup of hot water for 10-15 minutes. Tinctures are made by soaking the dried roots in alcohol or glycerin for several weeks. Capsules containing valerian root extract are also available and can be taken orally.

Storage: Dried valerian root should be stored in an airtight container in a cool, dark place to maintain its potency. Tinctures and capsules should also be stored in a cool, dry place.

Dosage: The valerian root dosage depends on the form it takes. As tea, 1-2 teaspoons of dried root can be steeped in a cup of hot water and consumed up to three times daily. Tinctures can be taken in drops, with a typical dose ranging from 20-30 drops up to three times daily. Capsules typically contain 300-500mg of valerian root extract and can be taken up to three times daily.

Benefits: Valerian root has been traditionally used as a natural remedy for anxiety and insomnia. Research has shown that valerian root can increase GABA (gamma-amino-butyric acid) levels in the brain, calming and helping alleviate anxiety. Studies have also demonstrated valerian root can improve sleep quality and reduce the time it takes to fall asleep. Additionally, valerian root has been shown to have anti-inflammatory and antispasmodic properties, making it potentially useful for conditions such as menstrual cramps and digestive issues.

Precautions: Valerian root is generally considered safe when taken as directed. However, it can cause drowsiness and should not be taken before driving or operating heavy machinery. Valerian root can also interact with certain medications, including sedatives and antidepressants. Individuals with liver disease, pregnant, or breastfeeding should consult a healthcare provider before using valerian root. Additionally, valerian root should only be used consecutively for up to two weeks without consulting a healthcare provider.

Conclusion: Valerian root is a natural pain reliever used for centuries due to its sedative and anxiolytic effects. It can be prepared in various ways, including as a tea, tincture, or capsule. Valerian root effectively reduces anxiety, improves sleep quality, and relieves pain. However, precautions should be taken when using valerian root, and it is essential to consult with a healthcare provider before using it as a treatment for any specific condition.

Valerian Root Coffee

Method of drying and roasting valerian root to make ground coffee:

Valerian has a distinctive smell and taste that some people find unappealing. Mix it with regular coffee or roasted root (like chicory) to make it more palatable. It is also very potent, so start with a small amount and adjust to taste. It is also known for its sedative effects, so it's best to enjoy this drink when you're in for a relaxing day or winding down in the evening. Always consult a healthcare provider before starting any new supplement regimen, including valerian root, as it can interact with certain medications and may cause side effects in some individuals.

Drying Valerian Root

Harvest your valerian root: Valerian root is harvested in the autumn from plants at least two years old. After digging up your plant, shake off any excess soil and gently wash the roots.

Slice the roots: To allow them to dry more quickly and evenly, slice the roots into thin, uniform pieces.

Dry the roots: Lay out your sliced roots in a single layer on a drying rack, ensuring good airflow. Place the rack in a dry, warm, and dark location with good ventilation. This could be an airing cupboard, a loft, or a room with a dehumidifier.

Wait and turn: The drying process may take up to two weeks, depending on the thickness of your slices and the conditions in your drying location. Turn the slices every few days to ensure they dry evenly.

Check for dryness: The roots are sufficiently dry when they snap rather than bend. Once they reach this stage, they can be stored in an airtight container until you're ready to roast them.

Roasting and Grinding Valerian Root

Preheat your oven: Preheat your oven to around 225 degrees Fahrenheit (105 degrees Celsius).

Roast the roots: Spread your dried valerian slices on a baking sheet and place them in the oven.

Check regularly: Roasting times will vary based on your oven and the size of your root slices. Check the roots every 10 minutes to ensure they don't burn. You're aiming for a dark brown colour similar to roasted coffee, which may take 20-30 minutes.

Let them cool: Once roasted, remove the roots from the oven and allow them to cool.

Grind the roots: When the roasted roots are cool, they can be ground. A coffee grinder works well for this purpose. For use in a coffee maker, grind them to a similar consistency as coffee grounds.

Remember, valerian has potent effects and should be used sparingly.

Wood Avens (Geum urbanum)

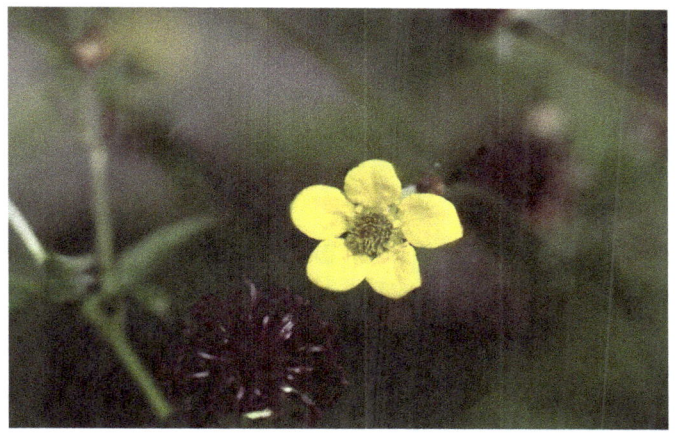

Wood Avens, also known as Herb Bennet or Colewort, is a perennial plant native to the U.K. and other parts of Europe. It has a rich history of traditional use for relieving various types of pain, including toothaches and stomach pain.

Harvesting: Wood Avens are harvested in the late spring to early summer when the plant is in bloom. Snip off the flowering tops, leaves, and roots. Be respectful to the plant and its surrounding environment, ensuring you do not overharvest and leave enough plant material for regeneration.

Preparation and Storage: After harvesting, wash the plant parts thoroughly and allow them to dry completely in a shaded, well-ventilated area. Once dried, the plant should be stored in an airtight container in a cool, dark place. Wood Avens can be prepared as a tea by steeping the dried plant parts in hot water.

Dosage and Precautions: Dosage can vary, but generally, tea is made by steeping one teaspoon of dried Wood Avens in a cup of hot water for 10-15 minutes. It is advised to start with a low dose to observe your body's reaction. Pregnant or breastfeeding women, children, and individuals with any medical condition should consult a healthcare professional before using Wood Avens.

Benefits and Mechanism of Action: Wood Avens contains tannins, eugenol, and other compounds with analgesic (pain-relieving) and anti-inflammatory properties. Eugenol, in particular, is known for its anaesthetic effects, which may help relieve toothaches.

Safety and Side Effects: Wood Avens is generally considered safe when used in moderation. However, excessive consumption may cause gastrointestinal issues such as nausea and diarrhoea. If you experience any adverse reactions, discontinue use and seek medical attention.

Conclusion: Wood Avens is a valuable natural analgesic that can be harvested and used to prepare herbal remedies for pain relief. Proper harvesting, preparation, and dosage ensure its efficacy and safety. As with all herbal treatments, it is essential to approach their use with care and consult a healthcare professional, especially if you have any health concerns or are taking other medications.

Interesting Fact: An interesting fact about Wood Avens is that people of the Middle Ages used it to ward off evil spirits and protect against venomous beasts.

Scientific Study: It's important to note that while there's historical and anecdotal evidence supporting the analgesic benefits of Wood Avens, comprehensive clinical studies are still limited. The presence of eugenol, a known natural anaesthetic, does lend credence to its traditional use for toothaches. Nevertheless, scientific research and clinical trials are needed to substantiate these claims and understand the full extent of Wood Avens' analgesic effects and other health benefits.

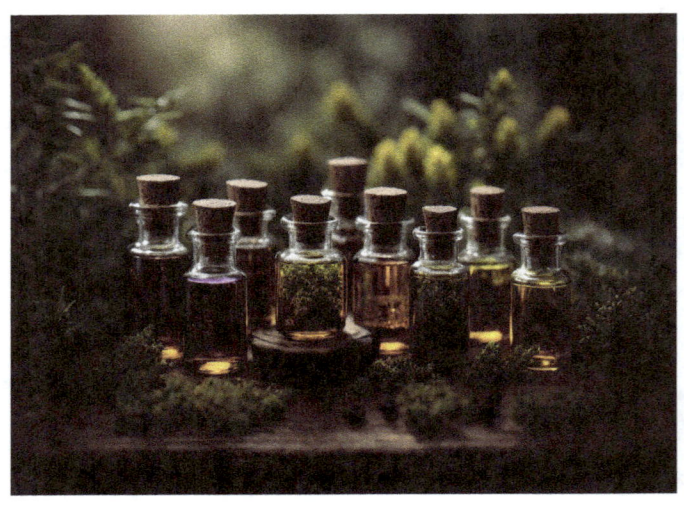

Lesser Celandine (Ficaria verna)

Lesser Celandine, native to the U.K., is a low-growing perennial herb recognised by its bright yellow flowers that bloom in early spring. Care should be taken despite its beauty, as all plant parts are toxic if ingested in large quantities.

Harvesting: For medicinal use, the roots of Lesser Celandine are typically harvested. The best time to do so is late autumn or early spring, when the plant's nutrients are most concentrated in the roots. Use gloves while handling to prevent skin irritation, and use a garden fork or spade to unearth the roots gently.

Preparation and Storage: After harvesting, clean the roots thoroughly and let them dry in a cool, dark, and well-ventilated area. Once dried, they can be ground into a powder for easy use. Store the dried or powdered roots in airtight containers in a cool, dark place for optimal preservation.

Dosage and Precautions: Ingestion is not advised due to toxicity. Use with caution in topical or transdermal application. Pregnant or breastfeeding women, children, and individuals with medical conditions should avoid Lesser Celandine unless under the supervision of a healthcare provider.

Benefits and Mechanism of Action: Historically, Lesser Celandine was used to alleviate haemorrhoid pain and discomfort, attributed to its anti-inflammatory properties. More scientific research is required to understand the exact mechanism of action.

Safety and Side Effects: Lesser Celandine should be approached cautiously due to its toxicity. Ingesting the plant may cause vomiting, diarrhoea, and abdominal pain. Topical use may also cause skin irritation in some individuals.

Conclusion: While Lesser Celandine has historical uses as a natural analgesic for specific conditions, its toxicity and potential side effects make it essential for individuals to use it cautiously. Adequate consultation with a herbalist or healthcare provider is necessary to ensure safe and effective use.

Interesting Fact: Lesser Celandine was one of the favourite flowers of the famous poet William Wordsworth, and he wrote three poems about the flower, celebrating its beauty.

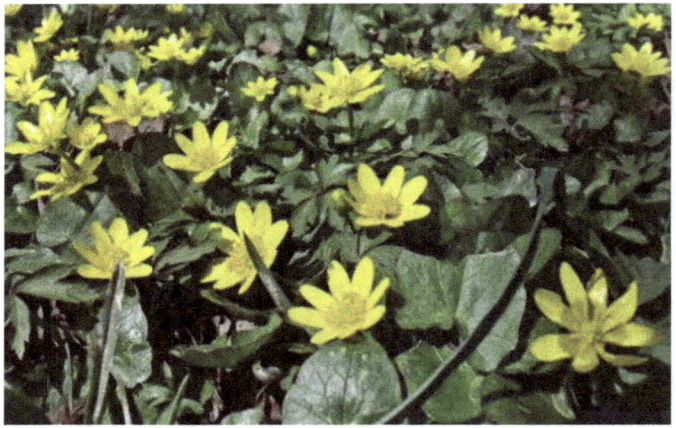

Lesser Celandine

Scientific Study: There is limited scientific research on the analgesic properties of Lesser Celandine. Most available studies focus on its toxic properties and effects on livestock and humans when ingested. Because of the scarcity of research on its medicinal benefits, extensive clinical studies and trials are required to establish the plant's safety and efficacy as a natural analgesic.

Note: This information is a general guide and does not substitute professional medical advice and treatment. It is crucial to consult healthcare professionals and exercise caution when using Lesser Celandine, considering its known toxicity and limited scientific backing for medicinal use.

Ingestion is not advised due to toxicity.

When it comes to herbal preparations, determining an exact dosage for topical application can be challenging, especially for plants like Lesser Celandine, where scientific research and evidence are limited. Furthermore, the plant's potential toxicity makes it essential to proceed cautiously.

Here's a generic guide that might help in preparing a topical application, but it's crucial to carry out a patch test to ensure no adverse or allergic reactions occur:

Preparing Lesser Celandine Topical Application

Dried Lesser Celandine Root Powder: Obtain the dried and powdered roots of Lesser Celandine. Ensure the roots have been cleaned and prepared correctly to avoid contaminants.

Base: Choose a base for your topical application. Coconut oil, almond oil, or an unscented lotion are good choices. The base will dilute the Lesser Celandine root powder and aid in application.

Mixing: Mix a small amount of the Lesser Celandine root powder with the base. Start with a low concentration (one teaspoon of root powder to four teaspoons of base) to minimise the risk of irritation. Mix the ingredients thoroughly until you achieve a smooth, consistent paste.

Patch Test: Before completing an application, apply a small amount of the mixture to a discreet skin area. Wait for 24-48 hours to observe if any adverse reactions (redness, itching, irritation) occur.

Application: Apply the mixture to the affected area if the patch test shows no adverse reactions. Apply a thin layer to the skin, massaging it in gently.

Frequency: Use sparingly, and monitor the skin for any reactions. If irritation occurs, wash the area thoroughly with soap and water and discontinue use.

Storage: Store any unused mixture in a cool, dark place. As with all natural preparations, use within a short period to ensure potency and safety.

Important Precautions: Consult a healthcare provider or experienced herbalist before using Lesser Celandine topically to ensure it's appropriate for your condition and won't interact with other treatments or medications you might be using.

Given the potential toxicity of Lesser Celandine, it's paramount to proceed with caution and prioritise safety in its use.

Note: This preparation guideline is general and does not guarantee safety or efficacy. Individual responses to herbal preparations can vary, and proper medical guidance is essential to ensure safe use.

Lesser Mugwort (Artemisia vulgaris)

Lesser Mugwort, known as common wormwood or wild wormwood, is a plant native to the U.K. and other parts of Europe and Asia. It has been traditionally used as a medicinal herb for various ailments, including pain and inflammation.

Harvesting: Lesser Mugwort is best harvested when the plant is fully blooming in late summer. Choose a dry, sunny day to gather. Cut the upper parts of the plant, including leaves and flowering tops, using sharp, clean scissors or pruners. Ensure sustainable harvesting by leaving enough plant material for regeneration.

Preparation and Storage: After harvesting, rinse the harvested parts thoroughly and dry them in a shaded, well-ventilated area. Once dried, the plant material can be stored in airtight containers in a cool, dark place for up to a year. Lesser Mugwort can make teas, tinctures, or salves for topical application.

Dosage and Precautions: As a general guideline, Lesser Mugwort tea can be prepared by steeping one teaspoon of dried herbs in a cup of hot water for 5-10 minutes. Pregnant and breastfeeding women and individuals with allergies to plants in the Asteraceae family should avoid Lesser Mugwort.

Benefits and Mechanism of Action: Lesser Mugwort contains various bioactive compounds, including volatile oils, flavonoids, and triterpenes, which may contribute to its anti-inflammatory and analgesic properties. These compounds can help reduce inflammation and alleviate pain.

Safety and Side Effects: Use Lesser Mugwort with caution as it can cause allergic reactions in individuals sensitive to plants in the Asteraceae family. Ingesting high doses may lead to gastrointestinal discomfort, including nausea, vomiting, and diarrhoea.

Conclusion: Lesser Mugwort is a traditional herbal remedy with potential analgesic and anti-inflammatory properties. Proper harvesting, preparation, and dosage are crucial for its safe and effective use.

As with all herbal treatments, consulting a healthcare professional or experienced herbalist is essential to determine the appropriate use and dosage.

Scientific Study: Comprehensive scientific studies regarding the analgesic effects of Lesser Mugwort are limited. A study published in the Journal of Ethnopharmacology (2014) highlighted the anti-inflammatory and pain-relieving effects of Artemisia species, which could be attributed to their flavonoid content. However, more rigorous clinical trials and research are needed to confirm Lesser Mugwort's analgesic benefits and safety.

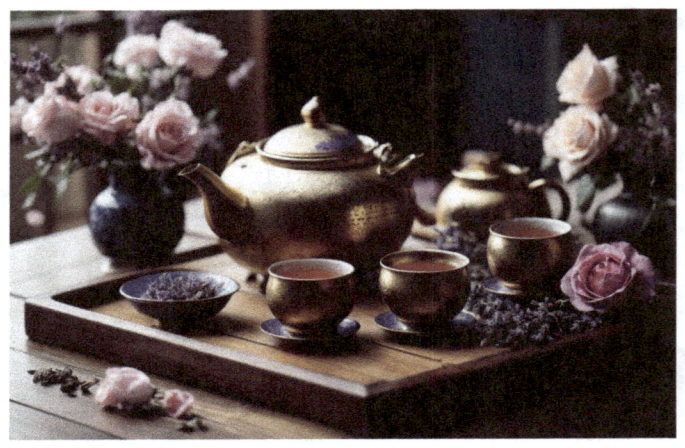

Medicinal Tea

"Trees are poems that the earth writes upon the sky." - Kahlil Gibran

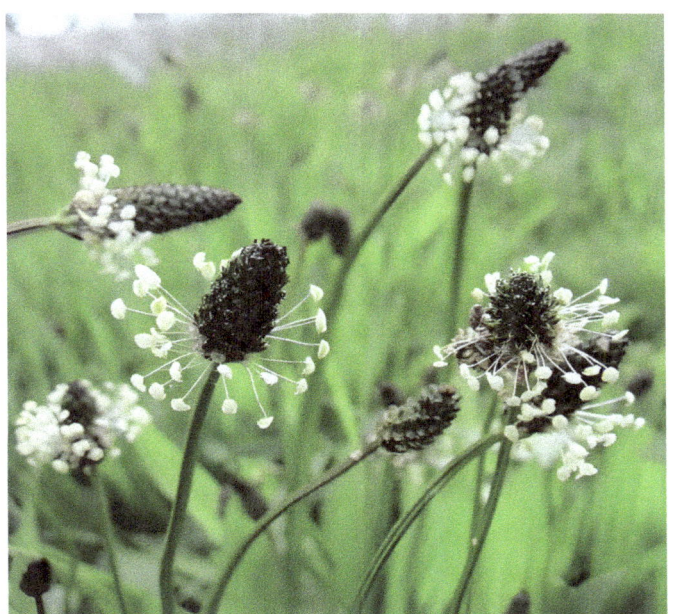

Plantain

Lesser Ribwort Plantain (Plantago lanceolata)

Lesser Ribwort Plantain is a perennial herbaceous plant native to the U.K. and Europe. Ribwort is known for its medicinal properties, and it has been used traditionally to treat various ailments, including pain and inflammation.

Harvesting: The best time to harvest Lesser Ribwort Plantain is in the late spring to early summer when the plant is flowering. Use clean, sharp scissors to cut the leaves and flowering spikes. As with wild harvesting, ensure sustainable harvesting practices, leaving enough plants for regeneration and local wildlife.

Preparation and Storage: After harvesting, clean the leaves thoroughly and allow them to dry in a well-ventilated, shaded area. The dried plant material can be stored in airtight containers in a cool, dark place for up to a year. Lesser Ribwort Plantain makes teas, infusions, or poultices for external application.

Dosage and Precautions: Dosage can vary, but generally, a tea can be made by steeping one teaspoon of dried Lesser Ribwort Plantain in a cup of hot water for 10-15 minutes. Pregnant and breastfeeding women and individuals with medical conditions should consult a healthcare professional before using this herb.

Benefits and Mechanism of Action: Lesser Ribwort Plantain contains various bioactive compounds, including flavonoids, terpenoids, and tannins, with anti-inflammatory and analgesic properties. It may help reduce inflammation and alleviate pain, though the precise mechanisms still need to be fully understood.

Safety and Side Effects: Lesser Ribwort Plantain is generally considered safe when used in moderation. However, some individuals may experience allergic reactions, particularly those allergic to plants in the Plantaginaceae family. Doing a patch test before using any plant-based topical preparation is always advised.

Conclusion: Lesser Ribwort Plantain is a valuable herb with a history of traditional use for relieving pain and inflammation. Proper harvesting, preparation, and dosage are essential for ensuring its efficacy and safety.

Interesting Fact: An interesting historical note is that Lesser Ribwort Plantain was referred to as the "soldier's herb" because of its use on the battlefield to promote wound healing.

Scientific Study: Although specific research on Lesser Ribwort Plantain's analgesic effects is limited, a study published in "The Journal of Ethnopharmacology" (2000) on another species of Plantago (Plantago major) showed significant wound-healing and anti-inflammatory properties, highlighting the potential of Plantago species, including Lesser Ribwort Plantain, in managing pain and inflammation. However, further scientific research and clinical trials are essential to confirm these properties and determine the optimal dosage and preparation methods.

Note: The above information is a general guide and does not substitute professional medical advice and treatment. Considering the limited scientific backing for its medicinal use, it's crucial to consult healthcare professionals and exercise caution when using Lesser Ribwort Plantain.

Couch Grass (Elymus repens)

Couch Grass, a perennial grass native to most of Europe, including the U.K., has been utilised traditionally for its medicinal properties. Though often seen as a weed, it has a long history of use for various ailments, including urinary tract infections and inflammation.

Harvesting: Couch Grass rhizomes (underground stems) are used primarily for herbal preparations. Couch Grass is ready to be harvested in the spring or autumn. Dig carefully around the plant to expose the rhizomes, then cut or gently pull them from the soil, ensuring they remain intact as much as possible.

Preparation and Storage: After harvesting, wash the rhizomes thoroughly and allow them to dry completely in a cool, dark, well-ventilated area. Once dried, the rhizomes can be chopped or ground and stored in an airtight container in a cool, dark place for up to a year.

Dosage and Precautions: A general dosage recommendation for Couch Grass is to steep 1-2 teaspoons of dried rhizome in a cup of boiling water for 10-15 minutes to make a tea. Pregnant or breastfeeding women and individuals with allergies should exercise caution.

Benefits and Mechanism of Action: Couch Grass contains compounds such as polysaccharides, saponins, and mucilage, which may contribute to its anti-inflammatory properties. These components may help soothe irritated mucous membranes, particularly in the urinary tract, and help alleviate inflammation and pain.

Safety and Side Effects: Couch Grass is generally considered safe when used in moderation. However, allergic reactions may occur, especially in individuals allergic to grasses. Possible side effects include mild gastrointestinal upset.

Conclusion: Couch Grass is used for its anti-inflammatory and diuretic properties. Proper consultation, harvesting, and preparation are crucial to ensure safety and effectiveness.

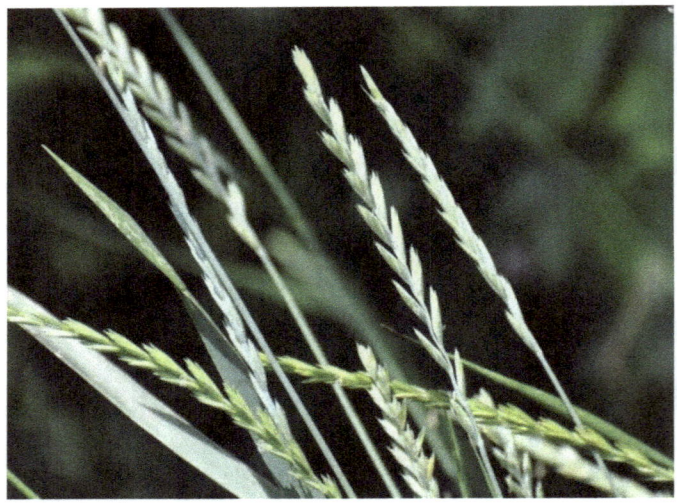

Couch Grass

Interesting Fact: Couch Grass has been used historically for medicinal purposes and as a source of food and fodder, demonstrating its versatility and importance in various cultures.

Scientific Study: Though specific research on Couch Grass's analgesic effects is limited, a study published in the journal "Phytomedicine" (2012) highlighted the anti-inflammatory effects of a related plant species (wheatgrass, Triticum aestivum). While not directly about Couch Grass, this study indicates the potential of grasses to reduce inflammation, which is often associated with pain.

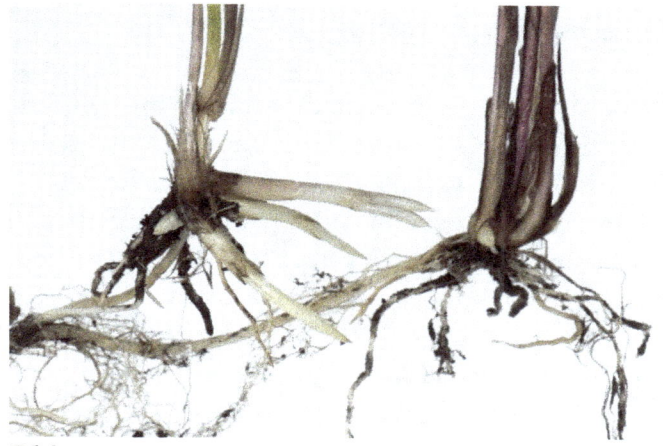

Rhizomes

Cowslip (Primula veris)

Cowslip is a perennial flowering plant native to the U.K. and other parts of Europe. It is significant in traditional medicine. It is often utilised for its anti-inflammatory and analgesic properties, particularly in treating joint pain and headaches.

Harvesting: Cowslip flowers are typically harvested in the spring when fully bloomed. It's crucial to pick the flowers gently without damaging the rest of the plant. Leaves can be harvested in the spring and autumn, and the roots in the autumn. As always, ensure sustainable harvesting practices.

Preparation and Storage: After harvesting, gently wash the flowers, leaves, or roots and dry them in a cool, dark, well-ventilated place. The dried parts can be stored in airtight containers in a cool, dark environment for up to a year. They can be used to make teas, tinctures, or topical salves.

Dosage and Precautions: For making cowslip tea, use one teaspoon of dried flowers steeped in a cup of boiling water for 10-15 minutes.

Pregnant or breastfeeding women and individuals allergic to plants in the Primulaceae family should avoid Cowslip.

Benefits and Mechanism of Action: Cowslip contains various compounds, including triterpenoid saponins and flavonoids, which have anti-inflammatory and analgesic effects. These compounds may reduce inflammation, thereby helping to alleviate pain.

Safety and Side Effects: Cowslip is generally considered safe when used in moderation. However, it may cause side effects in some individuals, including allergic reactions and gastrointestinal upset. It's always advised to perform a patch test before topical herbal preparations.

Conclusion: Cowslip is a traditional remedy with analgesic and anti-inflammatory properties. Specific scientific studies on Cowslip's analgesic properties are limited. However, a study published in "The Journal of Ethnopharmacology" (2009) reported the analgesic and anti-inflammatory effects of Primula veris (Cowslip) extract in experimental models, suggesting its potential for pain relief and anti-inflammatory effects.

Nettle (Urtica dioica)

Nettle, or stinging nettle, is a common plant in the U.K. renowned for its range of health benefits, including analgesic properties. Rich in various nutrients and compounds, nettle can be a versatile addition to herbal remedies.

Harvesting: The young leaves of the nettle plant are harvested, typically in the spring or early summer when the plant is most tender. Use gloves to avoid stinging and snip the top one-third of the plant with scissors or garden shears.

Preparation and Storage: Rinse nettle leaves under cold water to remove dirt and debris. To deactivate the stinging hairs, dry the leaves in an oven at a low temperature or air dry in a shaded, well-ventilated area. Once dried, store them in an airtight container in a cool, dark place. Dried nettles can be used to make tea tinctures or used in cooking.

Dosage and Precautions: To prepare nettle tea, steep 1 to 2 teaspoons of dried nettle leaves in hot water for 5 to 10 minutes. Adjust the dosage based on individual tolerance, and always consult a healthcare professional for personalised guidance.

Exercise caution, especially in pregnant or breastfeeding women, as excessive consumption can be harmful.

Benefits and Mechanism of Action: Nettle contains various compounds, such as polyphenols and flavonoids, which may have anti-inflammatory and analgesic properties. It's believed to help reduce the production of inflammatory chemicals in the body, relieving pain and inflammation.

Safety and Side Effects: Nettle is generally safe for most people when used in moderate amounts, but it can cause mild side effects, including digestive upset, skin irritation, and allergic reactions in some individuals. The stinging hairs on fresh nettle leaves can cause irritation and discomfort upon contact with the skin.

Conclusion: Nettle is a valuable plant with a long tradition of relieving pain and inflammation. Proper harvesting, preparation, and dosage are vital to ensuring its efficacy and safety.

Interesting Fact: Despite its stinging properties, nettle has been used in a process called urtication, where the fresh plant is deliberately applied to the skin to produce a stinging sensation, believed to relieve joint pain and arthritis symptoms.

Scientific Study: A study published in the "Journal of Ethnopharmacology" (2013) investigated stinging nettle's analgesic and anti-inflammatory properties. The research confirmed that nettle extracts could inhibit several key inflammatory events, contributing to its pain-relieving effects.

Hawthorn (Crataegus spp.)

Hawthorn, a well-recognised plant in the U.K., is notable for its heart health benefits. It has also been traditionally used to relieve pain, particularly chest pain associated with heart problems. Its berries, flowers, and leaves are all employed in natural medicine.

Harvesting: Hawthorn berries are generally harvested in the late summer to early autumn when fully ripened. The leaves and flowers are best gathered in the spring. Use garden shears or scissors for harvesting, ensuring it does not damage the plant.

Preparation and Storage: Clean the harvested parts gently and let them air-dry in a cool, well-ventilated area away from direct sunlight. Once dried, store in airtight containers in a cool, dark place. They can be used to make teas, tinctures, or extracts.

Dosage and Precautions: The typical dosage for Hawthorn (in tea form) is 1 to 2 teaspoons of dried leaves or berries steeped in hot water for about 15 minutes.

Benefits and Mechanism of Action: Hawthorn contains flavonoids and oligomeric procyanidins with antioxidant and anti-inflammatory properties. It is believed to improve blood flow, regulate blood pressure, and reduce inflammation, which can indirectly aid in relieving pain associated with heart conditions and improve overall heart health.

Safety and Side Effects: Hawthorn is generally considered safe, but side effects like dizziness, nausea, and digestive upset may occur. It can interact with certain heart medications.

Conclusion: Hawthorn is a promising remedy for heart health and related pain relief, demonstrating anti-inflammatory and antioxidant properties. Proper harvesting, preparation, and consultation with healthcare professionals ensure its beneficial use without adverse effects.

Interesting Fact: Hawthorn trees are often considered sacred in various cultures, believed to harbour fairies and provide protection and good fortune.

Scientific Study: A scientific study in the "Phytomedicine" journal (2010) explored the therapeutic properties of Hawthorn, including its anti-inflammatory effects. Reducing inflammation is crucial in pain management while not directly linked to the analgesic impacts. The research supports the traditional use of Hawthorn for heart health.

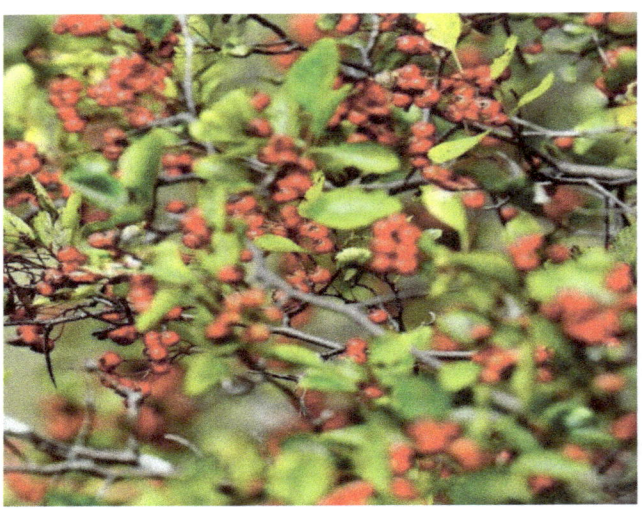

Hawthorn

Bog Myrtle (Myrica gale)

Bog Myrtle, a native plant in the U.K., Is traditionally used in natural medicine for its anti-inflammatory and analgesic properties. It has been used to address various ailments, including pain and inflammation.

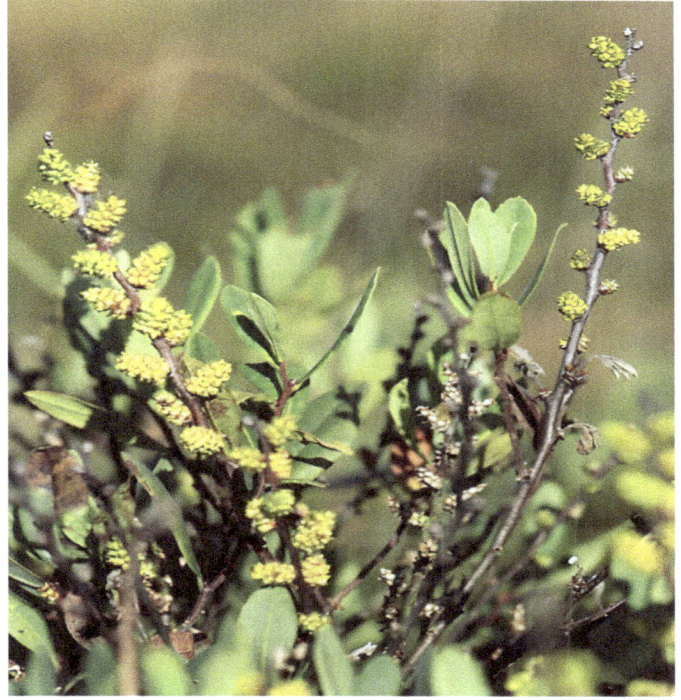

Bog Myrtle

Harvesting: Bog Myrtle leaves and flowers are harvested in late spring to early summer while they are most potent. Use scissors or pruning shears for harvesting, making clean cuts to avoid damaging the plant.

Preparation and Storage: Clean the harvested Bog Myrtle gently and let it air dry in a cool, dark, well-ventilated area. Once thoroughly dried, store the plant material in an airtight container in a cool, dark place for up to a year. The dried leaves can be used to make herbal teas or infused oils.

Dosage and Precautions: A typical dosage might be a cup of tea made from 1 teaspoon of dried Bog Myrtle leaves steeped in hot water for 10-15 minutes.

Benefits and Mechanism of Action: Bog Myrtle contains various compounds, including anti-inflammatory agents, which may help reduce inflammation and relieve pain.

Safety and Side Effects: While traditionally used, Bog Myrtle's safety profile for human consumption is poorly documented. Potential side effects and toxicity should be a concern.

Conclusion: With its traditional use as a natural remedy for pain and inflammation, Bog Myrtle holds promise. However, the lack of substantial scientific evidence regarding its efficacy, safety, and dosage warrants a careful and monitored approach to its use.

Interesting Fact: Bog Myrtle has been used historically as a natural insect repellent and is still used in some areas today.

Scientific Study: Scientific studies on Bog Myrtle are relatively scarce. A study published in "Phytotherapy Research" (2010) explored the anti-inflammatory properties of Myrica gale extracts, which may contribute to their analgesic effects. The study suggests potential anti-inflammatory effects, yet more comprehensive and human-focused research is crucial to confirm these findings and understand the implications for pain management.

Comfrey (Symphytum officinale)

Comfrey, known as knitbone, is a plant indigenous to the U.K., heralded for its healing properties. It alleviates pain, reduces inflammation, and accelerates the healing of bruises, sprains, and bone fractures.

Harvesting: For medicinal use, the leaves and roots of comfrey are harvested. The leaves are best harvested in late spring and early summer, while roots should be gathered in the autumn. Always use gloves and clean, sharp tools to cut the leaves or dig up the roots.

Preparation and Storage: Clean and dry the plant parts thoroughly in a well-ventilated, shaded area. Once dry, store in airtight containers in a cool, dark place. Comfrey can be used to make salves and oils.

Dosage and Precautions: Use sparingly and for a limited duration for topical applications such as salves and oils. Internal use is not recommended due to pyrrolizidine alkaloids, substances known to be harmful to the liver.

Benefits and Mechanism of Action: Comfrey contains allantoin, a compound that stimulates cell proliferation, aiding in healing broken bones, bruises, and sprains. The anti-inflammatory properties of comfrey contribute to pain reduction and improved healing.

Safety and Side Effects: While effective topically, comfrey is not advised for internal use due to pyrrolizidine alkaloids, which can cause liver damage and other serious health issues. It should be used cautiously and for short periods, even when used topically.

Conclusion: Comfrey stands out for its remarkable healing properties, particularly for bone and skin issues. Despite its benefits, careful handling and usage are essential to avoid potential health risks, and it is crucial to heed caution against internal use.

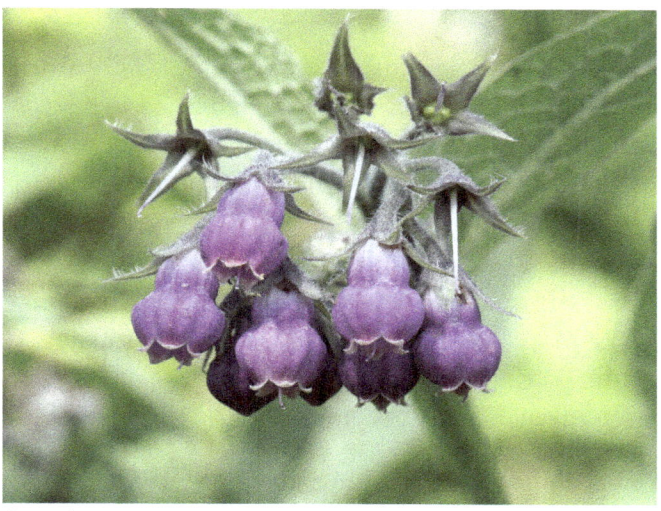

Comfrey

Interesting Fact: Historically, comfrey was so well-known for its bone-healing properties that it earned the nickname "knitbone."

Scientific Study: A study published in the "British Journal of Sports Medicine" (2012) examined the efficacy of comfrey root extract ointment in treating acute upper or lower back pain. The study found a significant reduction in pain intensity for participants treated with comfrey root extract, highlighting its potential as a natural pain-relieving topical treatment.

Feverfew (Tanacetum parthenium)

Feverfew, native to the U.K., is a popular natural remedy for managing fever, migraine headaches, and other ailments. Its delicate, daisy-like flowers and robust leaves are the main components used for medicinal purposes.

Harvesting: The leaves are typically harvested just as the plant comes into flower, generally in late spring or early summer. Snip the leaves off close to the stem using scissors or garden shears.

Preparation and Storage: After harvesting, wash the leaves gently and let them air dry in a cool, shaded area. Once dried, store the leaves in an airtight container in a dark, cool place. Feverfew can be used to make herbal teas or taken in capsule or tablet form.

Dosage and Precautions: The typical dosage of dried Feverfew for migraine prevention is around 50-150 mg daily. It is crucial to start with a lower dose to assess individual tolerance and consult a healthcare professional before use, particularly for individuals on blood-thinning medications or who are pregnant.

Benefits and Mechanism of Action: Feverfew contains a compound called parthenolide, which has anti-inflammatory and muscle-relaxant properties. These properties may contribute to its effectiveness in reducing the frequency and severity of migraine headaches by inhibiting the release of serotonin and prostaglandins, reducing inflammation and constriction of blood vessels in the brain.

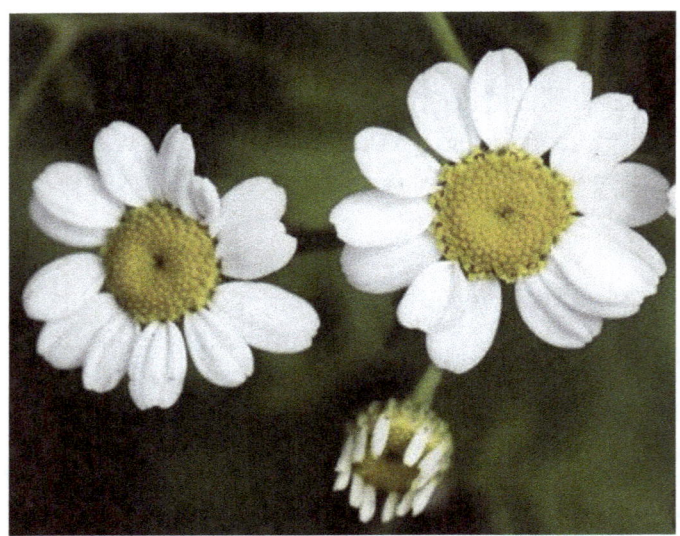

Feverfew

Safety and Side Effects: Generally considered safe when used appropriately, Feverfew may cause side effects such as mouth ulcers, digestive irritation, and increased risk of bleeding. It should be avoided by pregnant women and those on anticoagulant medications.

Conclusion: Feverfew is a promising herbal remedy for migraine prevention and overall pain reduction, thanks to its anti-inflammatory properties. However, appropriate dosage and adherence to safety precautions are imperative to ensure its beneficial use.

Interesting Fact: Despite its name, Feverfew was historically not the most popular herb for treating fevers; its name is derived from the Latin word "febrifugia," meaning "fever reducer."

Scientific Study: In a survey published in the British Medical Journal (1988), out of 270 people with migraines who used Feverfew daily as a prophylactic, 70% reported a reduction in the frequency and severity of migraine attacks. This study supports the anecdotal evidence and traditional use of Feverfew in migraine management, though more robust clinical trials are necessary to solidify these claims.

CHAPTER 11

Other Native Trees, Plants, and Fungi

with Painkilling Properties

In addition to the commonly known natural painkillers discussed in previous chapters, there are several other native trees, plants, and fungi in the United Kingdom that also possess painkilling properties. In this chapter, we will explore some of these lesser-known natural remedies.

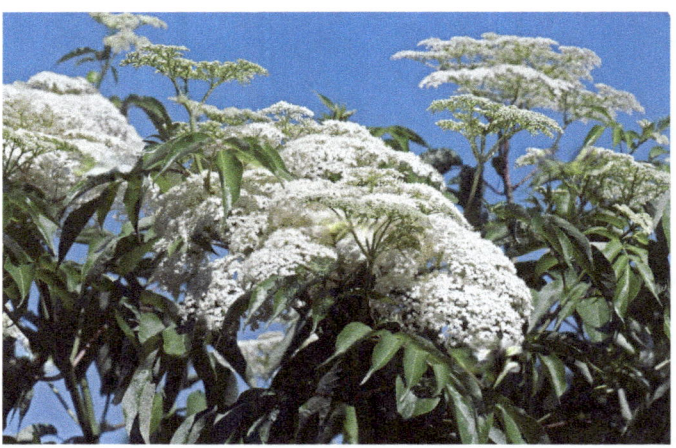

Elderflower

Elderflower is commonly found in hedgerows, woodlands, and along roadsides throughout the U.K. It has been traditionally used as a natural remedy for pain relief and inflammation, particularly for headaches and migraines. The flowers contain flavonoids and antioxidants that can help reduce inflammation and pain. They can be used fresh or dried and brewed as tea or added to a tincture.

Reishi mushroom is a fungus native to the U.K. and has been used in traditional Chinese medicine for thousands of years. It is known for its powerful anti-inflammatory and analgesic properties and is often used to treat pain associated with arthritis, fibromyalgia, and other chronic pain conditions. Reishi mushrooms can be brewed as tea, taken in capsule form, or used in a tincture.

Jewelweed, also known as touch-me-not, is a common plant that grows in damp areas throughout the U.K. It has been traditionally used to treat various ailments, including pain and inflammation. Jewelweed contains compounds called Lawsone and tannins, which have been shown to have anti-inflammatory and pain-relieving properties. The leaves and stems of jewelweed can be brewed as tea or made into a tincture.

Yarrow is a perennial herb that is native to the U.K. and is commonly found in meadows and grasslands. It has been traditionally used to treat pain and inflammation, particularly for menstrual cramps, headaches, and toothaches. The leaves and flowers of yarrow contain compounds called sesquiterpene lactones, which have anti-inflammatory and analgesic properties. Yarrow can be brewed as tea, or the leaves can be used to make a poultice.

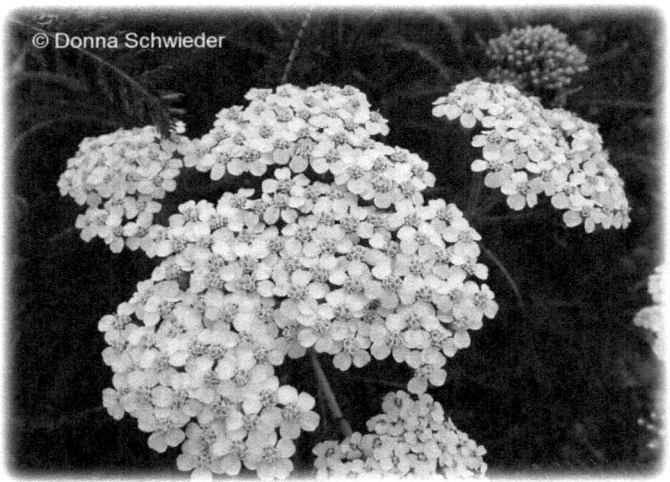

Yarrow

The horse chestnut is a tree that is native to the U.K. and is commonly found in parks and gardens. It has been traditionally used to treat pain and inflammation, particularly for conditions such as varicose veins and haemorrhoids. The bark and seeds of the horse chestnut tree contain a compound called aescin, which has been shown to have anti-inflammatory and analgesic properties. Horse chestnut can be brewed as tea, or the bark and seeds can be used to make a tincture.

Wild Lettuce is a plant that grows wild throughout the U.K. and has been traditionally used to treat pain and anxiety. It contains lactucarium, a natural compound that has analgesic and sedative properties. Wild Lettuce can be brewed as tea, or the leaves can be dried and smoked.

Some Interesting Facts about Smoking Wild Lettuce - and it's the medicinal use: Wild Lettuce is sometimes smoked for its medicinal properties, although this method is not standard. Smoking wild Lettuce is not the same as smoking cannabis, as wild Lettuce does not contain the psychoactive compound THC.

The mode of action of wild Lettuce within the body is poorly understood, but it is thought to have sedative and analgesic effects. In addition, some active compounds in wild Lettuce, such as lactucin and lactucopicrin, have been shown to have pain-relieving and calming effects in animal studies.

There are few clinical studies on the medicinal use of wild Lettuce, and more research is needed to understand its effects and potential benefits. One study published in the Journal of Ethnopharmacology in 2013 found that a wild lettuce extract had sedative effects in mice. Another study published in the same journal in 2014 found that a wild lettuce extract had a pain-relieving impact on rats.

In general, smoking any substance can adversely affect the lungs and overall health, and it is not a recommended method of administration for wild Lettuce or any other medicinal herb. However, wild Lettuce is commonly used in tinctures, teas, or capsules for its potential health benefits. As with any supplement or herb, speaking with a healthcare professional before using wild Lettuce is essential to ensure its safe and appropriate use.

19th Century: During the 19th Century in England, wild Lettuce, also known as Lactuca virosa, experienced a surge in popularity. It was used as an alternative to opium and was listed in the *British Pharmacopoeia. Physicians would use it as a sedative for conditions like insomnia and anxiety. It was also used to treat coughs and respiratory conditions, as it is thought to suppress coughs and aid in loosening and expelling phlegm.

*The British Pharmacopoeia (BP) is an authoritative, official collection of standards for U.K. medicinal substances. It is used by individuals and organisations involved in pharmaceutical research, development, manufacture, quality control, and analysis.

The first British Pharmacopoeia was published by the General Medical Council in 1864, consolidating several older publications and lists of medicines into a single, comprehensive document. This was part of an effort to standardise the production and use of medicinal substances.

The British Pharmacopoeia is updated annually to include new monographs and to revise existing ones to reflect advancements and changes in the medical and pharmaceutical industries.

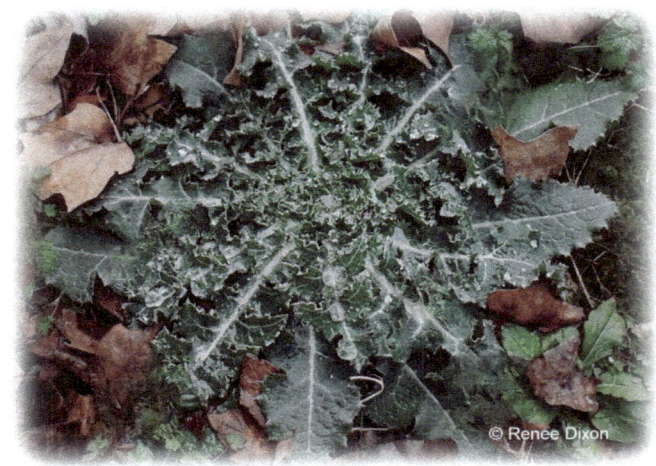

Wild Lettuce

"Nature alone is antique, and the oldest art a mushroom." - Thomas Carlyle

Quick recap

Birch Bark (Betula spp.): Birch Bark contains betulinic acid, known for its anti-inflammatory and skin-soothing properties, making it useful for various skin conditions and inflammatory disorders.

Bog Myrtle (Myrica gale): It is traditionally used as an insect repellent for skin conditions, owing to its essential oils and anti-inflammatory compounds.

Chanterelle Mushroom (Cantharellus cibarius): Beyond its nutritional richness, Chanterelle Mushrooms are a source of antioxidants and anti-inflammatory compounds, contributing to overall well-being.

Comfrey (Symphytum officinale): Allantoin in Comfrey aids in wound healing and has anti-inflammatory properties.

Couch Grass (Elymus repens): Couch Grass has historical usage for urinary tract and skin issues, attributed to its soothing polysaccharides.

Cowslip (Primula veris): The saponins present in Cowslip contribute to its sedative and anti-inflammatory properties.

Elderflower (Sambucus spp.): Elderflower is rich in flavonoids and has antiviral and immune-boosting properties.

Feverfew (Tanacetum parthenium): Parthenolide, a compound in Feverfew, helps reduce fever inflammation and prevent migraines.

Hawthorn (Crataegus spp.): Rich in flavonoids and oligomeric proanthocyanidins, Hawthorn supports heart health and provides anti-inflammatory benefits.

Horse Chestnut (Aesculus hippocastanum): Aescin, found in Horse Chestnut, supports vein health and reduces inflammation.

Jewelweed (Impatiens capensis): Jewelweed is often employed to alleviate skin irritations and rashes, thanks to its anti-inflammatory compounds.

Lavender Oil (Lavandula angustifolia): Linalool and linalyl acetate, primary components of lavender oil, are renowned for their anti-anxiety and calming effects, making it a preferred choice for stress relief and relaxation in aromatherapy.

Lesser Celandine (Ficaria verna): It has been used for its anti-haemorrhoidal properties, with its root tubers relieving haemorrhoids and skin issues.

Lesser Mugwort (Artemisia vulgaris): This plant has been employed for its digestive and anti-inflammatory benefits, with its essential oils potentially providing relief.

Lesser Ribwort Plantin (Plantago lanceolata): It offers anti-inflammatory and cough relieving properties, with its polysaccharides and antioxidants contributing to these effects.

Meadowsweet (Filipendula ulmaria): Meadowsweet contains salicylates and flavonoids, contributing to its anti-inflammatory and analgesic properties. It has been traditionally used for managing fever, pain, and various inflammatory conditions.

Nettle (Urtica dioica): Nettle is abundant in minerals and vitamins and is employed for its anti-inflammatory and nutritional benefits.

Poppy (Papaver spp.): Poppies, particularly the opium poppy, contain alkaloids like morphine and codeine, potent analgesics for managing moderate to severe pain.

Reishi Mushroom (Ganoderma lucidum): Rich in triterpenoids and polysaccharides, Reishi mushroom offers immune-boosting and anti-cancer benefits.

St. John's Wort (Hypericum perforatum): St. John's Wort contains hypericin and hyperforin, compounds believed to have potent antidepressant and mood-regulating properties. It alleviates symptoms of depression, anxiety, and related conditions.

Valerian Root (Valeriana officinalis): Valerian Root is rich in valerenic acid, a compound known for its sedative effects, aiding sleep and reducing anxiety.

Wild Lettuce (Lactuca virosa): Historically used as a sedative and pain reliever, its lactucopicrin contributes to these effects.

Willow Bark (Salix spp.): Willow Bark is rich in salicin, which the body converts to salicylic acid, providing anti-inflammatory and analgesic effects.

This natural pain reliever has been used for centuries to alleviate aches, pains, and fever.

Wood Avens (Geum urbanum): Used in traditional herbal remedies, Wood Avens is believed to possess mild astringent and anti-inflammatory properties.

Yarrow (Achillea millefolium): Yarrow contains azulene, providing anti-inflammatory and wound-healing properties.

Each species carries within its botanical matrix a wealth of compounds, contributing to their diverse therapeutic potentials and offering an array of healthful benefits.

Natural painkillers have many potential clinical applications, including treating chronic and acute pain, anxiety, depression, and inflammatory conditions. While they are often considered a safer alternative to prescription opioids, it is vital to use them with caution and under the guidance of a healthcare professional. Further research is needed to fully understand the potential clinical applications of natural painkillers and ensure their safety and efficacy.

Ongoing research

Ongoing research in the U.K., on the effectiveness of natural remedies for various health conditions. The U.K. has a long tradition of using natural remedies, and there is growing interest in the scientific study of these remedies.

One example of ongoing research in the U.K. is the National Institute for Health Research (NIHR) Complementary and Alternative Medicine (CAM) Speciality, which funds research into natural remedies and other forms of complementary and alternative medicine. This speciality supports research on various conditions, including chronic pain, anxiety, and depression.

Another example is the Centre for Evidence-Based Complementary Medicine at the University of Exeter, which researches the effectiveness of natural remedies for various conditions. For example, the centre has published numerous studies on herbal medicine for irritable bowel syndrome, acupuncture for chronic pain, and mindfulness-based interventions for depression and anxiety.

There are also many individual researchers and research institutions in the U.K. researching natural remedies, including the University of Oxford, the University of Southampton, and the University of Bristol, among others.

Overall, there is a growing body of research in the U.K. and elsewhere on the effectiveness of natural remedies for various health conditions. This research is helping to inform clinical practice and improve patient outcomes.

Further Exploring the World of Medicinal

Plants and Fungi in the U.K.

The realm of medicinal plants and fungi is fascinating and crucial in the ongoing search for novel treatments and therapies in the medical field. The significance of Plant and Fungi in Medicine reveals that these natural entities have been pivotal in providing primary healthcare solutions, especially in pain management, for centuries. With its rich biodiversity, the U.K. has become a significant player in exploring the medicinal potentials of its native flora and fungi.

Kew Gardens: A Hub for Plant and Fungi Research

Delving into the lush and vibrant world of Kew Gardens, we find a plethora of information and research dedicated to plants and fungi. Research Focus and Achievements at Kew Gardens are notably extensive, covering various aspects from basic plant biology to the potential medicinal applications of native flora. Furthermore, accessing information from Kew Gardens is relatively straightforward, with their website being a treasure trove of data and their team being accessible for deeper inquiries.

Universities and Research Institutes

The U.K. has several esteemed universities with dedicated research programs focusing on medicinal plants and natural products. The University of Oxford and the University of Cambridge have been at the forefront, with numerous research projects exploring the therapeutic potentials of native flora. Similarly, the University of Edinburgh and Imperial College London have showcased significant contributions in the field, with their research often paving the way for discoveries and applications in medicine.

Royal Botanic Garden Edinburgh

Another beacon of plant research and conservation is the Royal Botanic Garden Edinburgh. Their Research and Conservation Efforts are nationally and globally recognised, contributing significantly to understanding plants and fungi. Moreover, their Collaborations and Discoveries with international organisations and researchers have broadened the horizons of plant-based medicinal research, providing new insights and possibilities in the field.

Pharmaceutical Companies and Clinical Trials

In the corporate world, numerous pharmaceutical companies are delving into the potential of natural compounds derived from native trees, plants, and fungi. Monitoring Research and Trials is essential to stay abreast of the latest developments and breakthroughs. Engaging with Ongoing Studies through various platforms, such as the U.K. Clinical Trials Gateway, can also provide valuable insights into the current research scenario and upcoming trials.

Exploring medicinal plants and fungi in the U.K. is a vast and ever-expanding field, intertwining various sectors from academic research institutes to pharmaceutical companies. The collective efforts from these entities not only enhance our understanding of the medicinal properties of native flora and fungi but also pave the way towards developing novel, effective treatments for various ailments, including pain management. Always remember, while the field is burgeoning with potential, consulting healthcare professionals and experts ensures that the information and applications are reliable and safe.

Further reading resources

Several published resources in the public domain provide information on the medicinal properties of native trees, plants, and fungi. Here are a few examples:

"**A Modern Herbal**" by Mrs. M. Grieve: Originally published in 1931, this classic herbal reference book provides detailed information on the medicinal uses of various plants, including many native to the U.K. It covers herbal remedies, plant folklore, and botanical descriptions. "A Modern Herbal" is available in the public domain and can be accessed online or downloaded as a PDF.

"**British Herbal Pharmacopoeia**" by the British Herbal Medicine Association: This publication offers a comprehensive guide to the therapeutic uses of herbal medicines, including those derived from native plants in the U.K. It provides detailed monographs on individual herbs, discussing their traditional benefits and indications. While the most recent edition is not available in the public domain, older versions from the 1980s and 1990s can be found online.

"**Medicinal Plants of the British Isles**" by C.F. Leyel: This book, first published in 1937, explores the medicinal properties of various plants found in the British Isles. It includes information on their historical uses, folklore, and traditional applications. While it may be challenging to find a physical copy, digital versions of "Medicinal Plants of the British Isles" can be accessed through various online platforms.

"**Flora of the British Isles**" by Clive Stace: Although not solely focused on medicinal properties, this botanical reference book provides extensive information on the native flora of the British Isles. It includes descriptions, illustrations, and distribution maps of numerous plant species, some of which may have medicinal uses. "Flora of the British Isles" is widely available in libraries and book-stores. These resources can serve as starting points for exploring the medicinal properties of native plants in the U.K. However, it is essential to note that scientific understanding and research have advanced since their publication. Consulting more recent scientific literature and research papers is recommended for up-to-date information.

Resources available via the public domain:

The Hathi Trust Digital Library is a large-scale collaborative repository of digital content from research libraries, which includes content digitised via Google Books and the Internet Archive, as well as digitised content of its own, offering an array of resources across numerous formats like books, journals, and government documents, with a mission to contribute to research, scholarship, and the common good by collaboratively collecting, organising, preserving, communicating, and sharing the record of human knowledge.
www.hathitrust.org

Project Gutenberg is one of the largest and oldest digital libraries, offering over 60,000 free eBooks. It includes many public-domain books, including classic literature, reference works, and non-fiction titles. www.gutenberg.org

Open Library is an online project that aims to create a web page for every published book. It provides access to various books, including public domain works, and allows users to borrow digital copies. www.openlibrary.org

Conclusion

For aeons, humanity has sought solace in nature's myriad elixirs to assuage anguish and malaise. The British Isles, replete with a bountiful miscellany of indigenous flora, timber, and mycological wonders, have been identified as reservoirs of analgesic virtues. From the venerable willow to the subtle meadowsweet, from the luminous chanterelle to the stoic birch, myriad natural concoctions beckon with promises of pain relief.

Yet, amidst the allure of these botanical panaceas, one must not succumb to the mirage of them being a pantheon for all ailments. Before embarking on a journey with nature's remedies, seeking counsel from those versed in the medical arts is sagacious.

Gathering nature's treasures demands both respect and circumspection. One must tread lightly, adhering to the code of ethical gleaning. Mastery over the arts of refinement, conservation, and quantification ensures both their potency and the safety of their embrace.

Woven judiciously into the tapestry of our existence, these botanical saviours promise relief and diminishing dependence on the synthesised potions of our age. Enriching meals with aromatic herbs, imbibing infusions steeped in healing, and anointing oneself with distilled essences represent but a smattering of modalities to usher these remedies into our quotidian.

The lure of nature's analgesics as a counterfoil to their pharmaceutical counterparts is undeniable. Yet, venturing into this realm demands prudence, soliciting expert guidance, and adhering to time-honoured protocols of gleaning, craft, and administration. In honouring these tenets, we harness the curative tapestry of the earth and journey towards a life marked by wellness and ecological harmony.

Glossary

2-arachidonoylglycerol (2-AG): An Endocannabinoid neurotransmitter that certain natural pain-relieving compounds might modulate.

Acetyl: A functional group present in various organic compounds that might be involved in the analgesic effects of plants and fungi.

Acute: Refers to sudden onset of typically severe pain, highlighting the importance of swift and effective pain relief, which natural remedies may provide.

Aglycone: The non-sugar component in a glycoside compound. Some aglycones in plants have potential analgesic effects.

Agropyrene: A compound present in certain plants like Couch Grass (Elymus repens), potentially contributing to their analgesic effects.

Alkaloids: A group of naturally occurring chemical compounds that mostly contain basic nitrogen atoms. They have a range of pharmaceutical effects and can be found in plants like poppy, which includes morphine, a potent alkaloid analgesic.

Allantoin: Present in comfrey, it aids in wound healing and has anti-inflammatory properties, relieving pain and discomfort.

Amide Hydrolase (FAAH): An enzyme that may be inhibited by certain natural compounds, leading to potential analgesic effects.

Analgesic: A term for drugs or other agents that can relieve pain, such as the salicin found in willow bark, which has analgesic properties.

Antagonist: A substance that interferes with or inhibits the physiological action of another, possibly used in pain management.

Antinociceptive: A term for substances that reduce sensitivity to painful stimuli, a property that might be found in certain plants and fungi.

Antioxidants: Compounds that may contribute to various plants and fungi' anti-inflammatory and analgesic effects.

Anxiolytic: Compounds like Linalyl acetate in Lavender Oil have anxiolytic properties, helping to reduce anxiety, which can aggravate pain perception.

Aryl: A functional group derived from an aromatic ring, possibly in compounds with analgesic properties.

Autotrophs: Organisms that produce food, including many plants that contain natural analgesics.

Benzene: A chemical compound present in specific natural remedies, contributing to their bioactive properties.

Benzene Ring: A hexagonal ring of carbon atoms potentially present in the molecular structure of natural analgesic compounds.

Beta-Caryophyllene: A dietary cannabinoid found in many essential oils from plants, potentially contributing to analgesic effects.

Beta-Glucans Polysaccharides: Found in the cell walls of certain fungi like Reishi Mushroom, possibly offering immunomodulatory and analgesic effects.

Betulin: Found in birch bark, betulin is a compound that has anti-inflammatory and skin-soothing properties.

Biodiversity: Refers to the variety of plant and fungi species in the U.K., many of which, like the meadowsweet and chanterelle mushroom, have painkilling properties.

Bioactive Compounds: Substances such as hypericin and hyperforin in St. John's Wort have a biological effect on the human body, often contributing to pain relief and healing.

Birch Bark: From the birch tree, birch bark contains betulin and other compounds that may act as analgesics or anti-inflammatory agents.

Bog Myrtle (Myrica gale): This plant is recognised for its pain relief and anti-inflammatory properties.

Brain-derived neurotrophic Factor (BDNF): A protein that certain natural compounds may modulate to provide neuroprotective and analgesic effects.

Camphor: A compound found in various plants, potentially offering analgesic and anti-inflammatory effects.

Carbon: A fundamental element in the chemical structure of natural analgesic compounds.

Cardiovascular: Relating to the heart and blood vessels, a system potentially affected by certain natural analgesic compounds.

Chanterelle Mushroom: A fungus with potential anti-inflammatory properties, contributing to its role in pain management.

Chemokines: A family of small cytokines or signalling proteins secreted by cells, potentially modulated by natural analgesics for anti-inflammatory effects.

Chronic: Refers to persistent, long-term pain that various natural analgesics may alleviate.

Cineole: A compound also known as eucalyptol, found in various plants and potentially offering analgesic and anti-inflammatory effects.

Codeine: A naturally occurring alkaloid found in the opium poppy, known for its analgesic properties.

Comfrey (Symphytum officinale): A plant that contains allantoin and other compounds, traditionally used for its anti-inflammatory and wound-healing properties.

Compounds: General term for chemical substances found in various plants and fungi, which contribute to their pain-relieving properties.

Coumarins: Phytochemicals that may have analgesic or anti-inflammatory effects in various plants.

Couch Grass (Elymus repens): A plant whose rhizomes may have analgesic and anti-inflammatory properties.

Cowslip (Primula veris): A plant used in traditional medicine, which may offer analgesic benefits.

Cyclooxygenase Enzymes: Enzymes that may be inhibited by certain natural compounds, leading to anti-inflammatory and analgesic effects.

Cytokines: Proteins that can influence inflammation and pain, potentially modulated by various natural remedies.

Decarboxylating: Decarboxylating refers to the chemical process of removing a carboxyl group from a molecule, often involving the release of carbon dioxide, which in the context of making a herbal salve, involves heating the herbs to activate certain therapeutic compounds before they are infused into the salve.

Deciduous: Refers to plants, like the birch tree, that shed their leaves annually, with various parts used for their analgesic or anti-inflammatory properties.

Diuretic: Substances like those found in nettle (Urtica dioica) increase urine production, potentially helping to eliminate toxins and reduce inflammation and pain.

Dopamine: A neurotransmitter that plays a role in pain perception and relief. Certain natural painkillers may impact dopamine levels to exert analgesic effects.

Elderflower: Used traditionally for its anti-inflammatory and pain-relieving properties, potentially linked to its bioactive compounds.

Endocannabinoids: Endogenous ligands that bind to cannabinoid receptors in the body, potentially influenced by certain natural analgesics for pain relief.

Endomycorrhizae: A symbiotic relationship between fungi and plant roots that may play a role in the plant's production of analgesic compounds.

Enzymes: Biological molecules that may be influenced by certain natural compounds, potentially contributing to analgesic and anti-inflammatory effects.

Ergosterol: A compound found in fungal cell membranes, such as in Reishi mushroom, potentially contributing to immunomodulatory and analgesic effects.

Essential Oils: Concentrated liquids containing volatile aroma compounds from plants, including Lavender Oil, which may have analgesic properties.

Esters: Chemical compounds derived from acids, potentially present in various plants and fungi with analgesic effects.

Ethnopharmacology: The study of the medicinal use of plants and fungi, particularly those with analgesic properties.

Eugenol: A compound found in various essential oils, potentially offering analgesic and anti-inflammatory effects.

Eukaryotes: Organisms with complex cells, including all plants and fungi, many of which produce natural analgesics.

Feverfew (Tanacetum parthenium): A plant containing parthenolide has anti-inflammatory and pain-relieving properties.

Flavonoids: Compounds found in various plants that may offer anti-inflammatory and analgesic benefits.

Free Radicals: Atoms or molecules that may be neutralised by antioxidants found in various plants and fungi, potentially contributing to analgesic and anti-inflammatory effects.

Fungi: Organisms like chanterelle and Reishi mushrooms are traditionally used for their potential analgesic properties.

Fusion: The process by which multiple entities combine, possibly relating to cellular processes in plants and fungi that produce analgesic compounds.

GABA-A: A receptor that, when activated, may have analgesic effects. Compounds in plants like Wild Lettuce may influence these receptors.

Gametes: Sex cells produced by many plants may be involved in the reproduction of plants growing natural analgesics.

Glioblastoma Cells: Cancer cells that certain natural compounds for analgesic and anti-cancer effects may target.

Glucose: A simple sugar that may be involved in the structure of glycosides found in various plants and fungi with potential analgesic properties.

Glycosides: Compounds found in various plants may have analgesic properties, such as those found in Willow Bark (containing salicin, a glycoside).

Gram-Positive: A type of bacteria that may be affected by compounds in certain plants, potentially related to the plants' anti-inflammatory or analgesic effects.

Hawthorn (Crataegus spp.): A plant with cardiovascular benefits, indirectly assisting pain management by enhancing overall health.

Hyperforin: A compound found in St. John's Wort with potential analgesic effects, possibly by impacting neurotransmitter activity.

Hypericin: A compound found in St. John's Wort, known for its potential analgesic and anti-inflammatory properties.

Hyphal: Pertaining to hyphae, the thread-like structures of fungi relevant to medicinal mushrooms like Reishi and Chanterelle.

Infusion: A method of extracting compounds from plants, which may be used to harness the pain-relieving properties of various herbs.

Iridoid Glycosides: Present in plants like Valerian Root, these compounds may contribute to the plants' analgesic effects.

Jewelweed: A plant traditionally used to relieve pain and inflammation, possibly due to various bioactive compounds.

Ketones: Organic compounds in some plants that may have a role in their analgesic properties.

Lactone: A type of molecule that may be found in certain plants and fungi, potentially contributing to their analgesic properties.

Lactucarium: A substance derived from Wild Lettuce, traditionally used for its sedative and pain-relieving properties.

Lactucin and Lactucopicrin: Compounds found in wild lettuce, potentially responsible for its purported pain-relieving effects.

Lavender Oil: An essential oil known for its calming effects and potential analgesic and anti-inflammatory properties.

Lesser Celandine (Ficaria verna): A plant traditionally used for its anti-inflammatory properties and potential to relieve pain.

Lesser Mugwort (Artemisia vulgaris): Traditionally used in herbal medicine for various ailments, including pain relief.

Lesser Ribwort Plantain (Plantago lanceolata): A medicinal herb potentially offering anti-inflammatory and analgesic properties.

Leukotrienes: Inflammatory molecules that certain natural analgesics may modulate.

Linalyl Acetate: is a compound in lavender oil, contributing to its potential analgesic effects.

Lupeol: is a natural compound found in various plants, possibly contributing to their analgesic and anti-inflammatory effects.

Meadowsweet: A plant that contains salicylic acid, an effective compound for pain and inflammation relief.

Meristematic Tissue: Consists of continuously dividing cells that generate new plant cells. It is located in areas of a plant where growth occurs such as the tips of roots, stems, and branches. The primary role of this tissue is to facilitate plant growth. Cells in meristematic tissue are typically small and cube-shaped.

Molecule: Pertains to the structure of various analgesic compounds found in the plant, tree, and fungi kingdom.

Monoacylglycerol Lipase (MAGL): An enzyme that may be influenced by certain plant compounds, affecting pain signalling pathways in the body.

Morphine: A potent analgesic compound naturally found in some plant species like the poppy.

Mucilage: A viscous secretion of some plants providing a soothing effect and potentially beneficial for pain relief.

Myrcene: A terpene found in many plants, known for its potential anti-inflammatory and analgesic properties.

Naphthodianthrone: Is a compound in St. John's Wort that contributes to the plant's potential analgesic effects.

Nettle (Urtica dioica): A plant with stinging hairs, used traditionally as a source of relief for various types of pain, possibly due to its different bioactive compounds.

Neurological: Pertaining to the nervous system, relevant in the context of neuropathic pain and the action of certain natural analgesics.

Neuropharmacology: The study of how drugs affect cellular function in the nervous system. Plants like Willow Bark and Meadowsweet have been subjects in this field for their potential analgesic effects.

Neuroprotective: Refers to the capacity of specific plant and fungal compounds to protect nerve cells from damage and degeneration.

Neurotransmitter: A substance, the levels or actions of which may be altered by natural analgesic compounds, affecting pain perception and signalling

Nitrogen: Is essential to plant growth and health and in synthesising many bioactive compounds with potential analgesic properties.

Norepinephrine: A neurotransmitter that can be affected by various natural compounds, impacting pain signalling and perception.

Nonsteroidal Anti-inflammatory Drugs (NSAIDs): A class of drugs that provides analgesic and anti-inflammatory effects without using steroids, similar to some compounds found in various plants.

Oligomeric Proanthocyanidins (OPCs):
Antioxidants found in plants like Hawthorn,
potentially offering anti-inflammatory and
analgesic benefits.

Opioids: A class of drugs that includes natural
substances like morphine from the Poppy plant,
used for their potent analgesic effects.

Organic: Pertaining to natural compounds,
including those in plants and fungi that may have
analgesic properties.

Phenol: A type of organic compound found in
various plants and essential oils, contributing to
their potential therapeutic effects.

Phloroglucinol: A compound found in certain
plants that may have analgesic or anti-spasmodic
effects.

Phytotherapy: Using plants for healing, including
plants with analgesic properties.

Polymer: Related to the structure of certain plant
compounds that may have therapeutic effects.

Polysaccharides: Found in various plants and fungi, these compounds may have immunomodulatory and other health-related effects.

Poppy: Known for containing morphine, a potent natural painkiller and the basis for many opioid medications.

Populus: Botanical name for the willow tree, a natural source of salicin, which may relieve pain and inflammation.

Precursor: A substance from which another is formed, primarily by metabolic reaction. For example, ranunculin is a precursor to protoanemonin in the body.

Primulaverin: A glycoside found in Cowslip (Primula veris), possibly contributing to the plant's potential analgesic properties.

Primverin: A compound found in certain plants like cowslip that may have health benefits.

Prostaglandins: Lipid compounds derived enzymatically from fatty acids, playing a role in inflammation and pain; their production is affected by various natural compounds.

Protoanemonin: A toxic compound found in some plants like lesser celandine, which has potential analgesic effects after being metabolised in the body.

Psychoactive: Is a term for substances that affect the mind, like certain compounds in Poppy.

Pyrrolizidine Alkaloids: Natural toxins found in certain plants that can cause liver damage. They should be avoided in plants used for analgesic purposes.

Ranunculin: A glucoside in Lesser Celandine may convert to analgesic protoanemonin in the body.

Reishi Mushroom: A fungus with potential immune-boosting and analgesic properties due to the presence of compounds like beta-glucans.

Rhizome: A type of underground stem found in Couch Grass (Elymus repens), which may have analgesic properties.

Salicin: Is a compound found in willow bark with analgesic and anti-inflammatory properties.

Salicylates: Chemical compounds found in plants like Meadowsweet, potentially offering analgesic and anti-inflammatory effects.

Salicylic Acid: An analgesic compound derived from various plants, including willow bark and Meadowsweet.

Salves: Topical applications from plant extracts for treating pain and other conditions.

Serotonin: A neurotransmitter that plays a role in pain perception, affected by various natural compounds.

St. John's Wort (Hypericum perforatum): A plant used traditionally for its many health benefits, including potential analgesic effects due to compounds like hypericin and hyperforin.

Substrate: The base on which fungi grow may contain natural analgesic compounds.

Synthetic: Refers to artificial compounds, in contrast to the natural analgesic compounds found in plants and fungi.

Tannins: Polyphenolic compounds found in Bog Myrtle (Myrica gale) and other plants, potentially contributing to analgesic effects.

Terpenes: A large group of volatile, unsaturated hydrocarbons found in the essential oils of plants, some of which have analgesic properties.

Terpinen-4-ol: A monoterpene alcohol found in Lavender Oil, possibly contributing to its analgesic and anti-inflammatory properties.

Thujone: A ketone and a monoterpene that exists in two stereoisomers: (+)-α-thujone and (−)-β-thujone. Found in Lesser Mugwort (Artemisia vulgaris), it may have analgesic properties.

Tinctures: Liquid extracts made from herbs that are taken orally and used for pain relief and other health benefits.

Topical: Referring to external application, many plants are used topically for pain relief and anti-inflammatory effects.

Valerian Root: A root used traditionally for its calming and analgesic effects, possibly due to various bioactive compounds.

Volatile: Compounds that quickly evaporate at normal temperatures, such as those found in essential oils of plants, some having analgesic properties.

Willow Bark: A natural source of salicin, offering potential analgesic and anti-inflammatory effects as a precursor to modern aspirin.

Wood Avens (Geum urbanum): A plant with anti-inflammatory and analgesic properties, potentially due to compounds like tannins.

Yarrow: A plant potentially offering analgesic and anti-inflammatory effects, possibly due to its diverse bioactive compounds.

"The best time to plant a tree was 20 years ago.
The second best time is now." -
Chinese Proverb

Bibliography

Books:

McIntyre, A., The Complete Herbal Tutor: The Ideal Companion for Study and Practice, (Aeon Books; Revised and Expanded edition April 2019).

Bruton-Seal, J. and Seal, M., Hedgerow Medicine: Harvest and Make Your Own Herbal Remedies, (Merlin Unwin Books; First Edition May 2008).

Easley, T. and Horne, S., The Modern Herbal Dispensary: A Medicine-Making Guide, (North Atlantic Books; 1st edition Nov. 2016).

Van Wyk, B.-E. and Wink, M., Medicinal Plants of the World, (CABI Publishing; 2nd Revised edition Jun. 2017).

White, L. B. and Foster, S., The Herbal Drugstore: The Best Natural Alternatives to Over-the-Counter and Prescription Medicines!, (Dutton / Signet; Illustrated edition April 2002).

Masé, G., The Wild Medicine Solution: Healing with Aromatic, Bitter, and Tonic Plants, (Healing Arts Press; Illustrated edition April 2013).

Chevallier, A., Encyclopedia of Herbal Medicine: 550 Herbs and Remedies for Common Ailments, (DK; 1st edition, July 2016).

Braun, L. and Cohen, M., Herbs and Natural Supplements, Volume 2: An Evidence-Based Guide, (Elsevier Health Sciences, 2015).

Benzie, I. F. F. and Wachtel-Galor, S., Herbal Medicine: Biomolecular and Clinical Aspects, Second Edition, (Boca Raton, CRC Press, 2011).

Blumenthal, M., The Complete German Commission E Monographs: Therapeutic Guide to Herbal Medicines, (Austin, American Botanical Council, 1998).

Tisserand, R. and Young, R., Essential Oil Safety: A Guide for Health Care Professionals, (Edinburgh, Elsevier, 2013).

Wood, M., The Practice of Traditional Western Herbalism: Basic Doctrine, Energetics, and Classification, (Berkeley, North Atlantic Books, 2004).

Hoffmann, D., Medical Herbalism: The Science and Practice of Herbal Medicine, (Rochester, Healing Arts Press, 2003).

Journal Articles:

Abdullah, M. Z. et al., 'Synthesis and Dehumidification Performance of Calcium Chloride Derived from the Waste Shells of Anadara Granosa', Applied Mechanics and Materials, 625 (2014).

Davis, E., 'The Treatment and Management of Chronic Pain Using CBD', (2020).

Handa, I. T. et al., 'Consequences of Biodiversity Loss for Litter Decomposition across Biomes', Nature, (2014).

Högberg, P. and Högberg, M. N., 'Does Successful Forest Regeneration Require the Nursing of Seedlings by Nurse Trees through Mycorrhizal Interconnections?', (2022).

Morris, R. S., 'Managed Realignment As a Tool for Compensatory Habitat Creation – A Re-appraisal', Ocean & Coastal Management, (2013).

Pereverzina, M., 'A Passive Constant Flow Regulator for Drug Delivery to the Human Lung in Portable Inhaler Systems', (2020).

Zia, Z., 'Synthesis and Characterisation of Low-cost Biopolymeric/Mineral Composite Systems and Evaluation of Their Potential Application for Heavy Metal Removal', (2022).

Webpages:

ADLERMECH. (n.d.) 'Lavender Essential Oil.' http://adlermech.com/tag/lavender-essential-oil/

Australian Car Sales. (2022) 'CBD and its interaction with the body.' http://australiancarsales.com/2022/shopping/cbd-and-its-interaction-with-the-body/

Blue Botanicals. (n.d.) 'CBD and the Endocannabinoid System: Unlocking the Secrets of How Our Bodies Heal and Thrive.' https://bluebotanicals.net/cbd-and-the-endocannabinoid-system-unlocking-the-secrets-of-how-our-bodies-heal-and-thrive/

Star Mushroom Farms. (n.d.) '4 Chicken Of The Woods Look Alikes.'
https://starmushroomfarms.com/chicken-of-the-woods-look-alikes/

Tripsitter. (n.d.) 'What Is the Endocannabinoid System?'
https://tripsitter.com/cannabis/endocannabinoid-system/

Online Published Studies:

Title: "Efficacy of Ginger for Alleviating the Symptoms of Primary Dysmenorrhea: A Systematic Review and Meta-analysis of Randomized Clinical Trials." Authors: Daily JW, Zhang X, Kim DS, Park S. Published: 2015
https://journals.plos.org/plosone/article?id=10.1371/journal.pone.0146211

Title: "Lavender and the Nervous System." Authors: Koulivand PH, Khaleghi Ghadiri M, Gorji A. Published: 2013
https://www.hindawi.com/journals/ecam/2013/681304/

Title: "Peppermint Oil for the Treatment of Irritable Bowel Syndrome: A Systematic Review and Meta-analysis." Authors: Khanna R, MacDonald JK, Levesque BG. Published: 2014
https://journals.lww.com/ibdjournal/Abstract/2014/07000/Peppermint_Oil_for_the_Treatment_of_Irritable_Bowel.13.aspx

Title: "Effect of Nigella sativa (black seed) on subjective feeling in patients with allergic diseases." Authors: Kalus U, Pruss A, Bystron J, Jurecka M, Smekalova A, Lichius JJ, Kiesewetter H. Published: 2003
https://pubmed.ncbi.nlm.nih.gov/14750201/

Title: "Analgesic and Anti-inflammatory Effects of Rosa damascena Hydroalcoholic Extract and its Essential Oil in Animal Models." Authors: Mahboubi M. Published: 2016
https://www.ncbi.nlm.nih.gov/pmc/articles/PMC4934652/

(Note: Some of the references do not have clear publication information available online, and thus are listed as "n.d." which stands for "no date".)

"To plant a garden is to believe in tomorrow." - Audrey Hepburn